SAND

Chief E.              , Refuge

# POWER
## AND
## CONTROL

Why charming men can make
dangerous lovers

3 5 7 9 10 8 6 4 2

Vermilion, an imprint of Ebury Publishing,
20 Vauxhall Bridge Road,
London SW1V 2SA

Vermilion is part of the Penguin Random House group of companies
whose addresses can be found at global.penguinrandomhouse.com

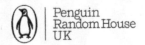

Penguin
Random House
UK

First published in 1991 by PAPERMAC as The Charm Syndrome
This edition published in 2017 by Vermilion

www.penguin.co.uk

A CIP catalogue record for this book is available from the British Library

ISBN 9781785041488

Typeset in India by Integra Software Services Pvt. Ltd, Pondicherry

Printed and bound by Clays Ltd, St Ives PLC

Penguin Random House is committed to a sustainable future for our
business, our readers and our planet. This book is made from Forest
Stewardship Council® certified paper.

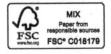

MIX
Paper from
responsible sources
FSC® C018179

# About the Author

Sandra Horley has been the Chief Executive of Refuge, the national domestic violence charity, since 1983. She has been working in the field of domestic violence for almost four decades, supporting women and children experiencing all forms of male violence and abuse.

Born in Ontario, Canada, Sandra read Sociology at McGill University in Montreal before coming to England, where she studied at the universities of Oxford and Birmingham. In 1979 she started working with abused and homeless women as director of the Haven project in Wolverhampton.

Sandra has acted as an expert witness in murder and manslaughter cases when the accused is an abused woman. She also directly supports families bereaved by domestic homicide. A committed campaigner on behalf of abused women and children, Sandra has not only played a pivotal role in raising the profile of domestic violence in the UK among the public, she has lobbied effectively for changes in government policy and legislation. She also advises governments internationally on gender-based violence and criminal justice.

Sandra has received prominent honours for her achievements in public life: a CBE in 2011 for 'services to the prevention of domestic violence' and an OBE in 1999 for 'services to the protection of women and children'. Under her leadership, Refuge was named Charity of the Year 2016 at the Charity Times Awards for its outstanding services and dedication to its clients in a difficult funding climate. Refuge currently supports almost 5,000 women and children on any given day.

Sandra has published two books on the subject of domestic violence and has written articles for the national press and professional journals. She also frequently gives talks and interviews. Sandra lives in London with her photographer husband, Julian Nieman, and has a daughter, Samantha Nieman.

He is
 charming,
  so,
   be sure
    that you
     keep him like fire
      beyond the tips of your fingers.
(Diane Wakoski, 'The Catalogue of Charms')

*For Julian and Sam.*

*In memory of my mother, who encouraged me
to challenge injustice.*

# Contents

# Acknowledgements

This book could not have been written without the contributions of many abused women who bravely shared their stories with me. To them my deepest gratitude. I would also like to thank the families I have worked with over the last decade who have lost loved ones to domestic violence. Their courage and strength in sharing their stories, so that others might be spared their agony, has made me more determined than ever to continue Refuge's work.

A very special thank you to Sheila Keating for working so hard on the first edition of this book. Her quick grasp of the material and her skill helped make the book a reality. Thanks to commissioning editor Katy Denny at Vermilion and editor Jane McIntosh for making the second edition happen, and to Lucy Snow at Refuge for her insight, intelligence and writing talent, and for supporting me with this edition. Thank you also to Elaine Hake for her immense contribution not only to this book but to the work of Refuge.

It would be impossible to name all of the amazing women and men who have been instrumental in championing the cause of domestic violence and pioneering the women's refuge movement – but I will give a special mention to Colin Brown, the late Neville Vincent and the late Lord Ashley. Without their dedication to the cause – as well as their personal support – Refuge would not be where it is today.

Various friends and Refuge colleagues have helped me by providing support, ideas and inspiration: you know who you are, but Jane Keeper, Ruth Aitken and Lisa King deserve a special mention for their tireless dedication to improving the lives of women and children. All of them have been selfless in their commitment to Refuge, and I appreciate their generous support and insight immensely. Together, we have achieved a huge amount. My gratitude also to Isobel Shirlaw and Julia Dwyer for supporting Refuge in its tenacious pursuit of justice for victims of domestic violence.

Thank you also to the many supporters, trustees and patrons who have supported Refuge's work over the years. Special thanks to Dame

Stella Rimington, who is a mentor and valuable sounding board and Maggie Rae, Refuge's fantastic chair. Thank you also to Baroness Helena Kennedy, QC, who champions women's rights and so frequently provides me with her wise counsel, and to Refuge patrons Cherie Booth QC and Sir Patrick Stewart. Patrick's unstinting support and courage in speaking out about his own experiences of domestic violence have been invaluable in raising the profile of Refuge, as well as much-needed funds. I am also grateful to my former assistant Pauline Persaud, who enabled me to deal with the demands of my work. Thanks to Nick Darke, Refuge's brilliant pro-bono designer, for his ongoing support and commitment.

Thank you to Elena and Helena Bonham Carter for their ongoing friendship. My gratitude also to Fred Mashaal for almost 40 years of friendship, encouragement and long-distance support. Without him, I would not be doing this work or have written this book. To Nancy, Harold and Martin Ship, and Don Kinder, for helping me in ways that have irrevocably changed my life for the better. And to Juergen Dankwort and Dr. Peter Jaffe, who have shaped and informed my thinking throughout my career.

Everything I do stems from my mother, the late Shirley Jane Horley, from her warmth, generosity, courage and remarkable spirit of survival. She taught me independence, belief in myself and to persevere against all odds.

There is no way I can adequately thank Aileen, my mother-in-law, who is now missed by us all, for her tireless loyalty and support. Her assistance was so often asked for and so freely given, from making curtains for our first refuge and answering the helpline, to providing a doting presence for Sam during those late-night crises at Refuge.

I am especially grateful to my husband, Julian, who has been consistently loving and supportive throughout my whole career, putting up with all those endless work phone calls. Not to mention the thousands of photographs he has generously taken to bring to life Refuge's work. Without him so much of what I have achieved would not have been possible.

To Sam, my daughter, who tolerated the closed door of my study for many years as a child and has grown into an amazing woman and trusted friend.

# Foreword by Sir Patrick Stewart OBE, Refuge Patron

I grew up in a home darkened by domestic violence. My father was an angry and unhappy man who used violence against my mother. As a child, I witnessed terrible things, but I felt powerless to stop the abuse.

In those days there was nowhere to go for help. Worse, there were those who allowed the abuse to continue. I heard police officers and ambulance-men standing in our small living room, saying things like '*She must have provoked him*' or '*Well, Mrs Stewart, it takes two to make a fight*'.

They had no idea. The truth is my mother did nothing to deserve the violence she endured. She did not provoke my father, and even if she had, violence is an unacceptable way of dealing with conflict. Violence is a choice a man makes and he alone is responsible for it.

When Sandra Horley asked me to become a patron of Refuge, back in 2007, I accepted without hesitation. I accepted for my mother. As a child, there was little I could do to help her. But as an adult, I can give support and encouragement to women who live in the same sort of fear that she did.

Of course, many things have changed since my mother's day. Since Refuge first opened its doors in 1971, it has grown to operate a national network of services that support thousands of women and children on any given day. It provides refuges across the country to keep women and children safe, advocates who protect women going through the courts, and runs countless other services that save and change lives.

But there is still a long way to go. The police often do not treat domestic violence with the seriousness it deserves. In my work with Refuge I have met families whose loved ones have been killed in terrible circumstances after the police failed to protect them.

The police had a duty to protect me and my mother, all those years ago, and they failed in that duty. It shocks me that, decades later, women and children are still being let down by those very agencies and professionals who are supposed to protect them.

This is why I am determined to carry on my work with Refuge. As well as providing vital services, Refuge campaigns tirelessly for improvements to the way the government and state bodies like the police and social services respond to vulnerable women and children. I am proud to support the efforts of this remarkable charity.

I know that many women may turn to this book in the hope of finding strength and peace. It is for them – and for my mother – that I continue to speak out against domestic violence and play my part in creating a world where women and children can live in safety, free from fear.

# Preface

I was prompted to write the first edition of this book in the early nineties by one woman in particular. A woman whose husband never hit her or even threatened to hit her but who made her life a living hell for 25 years. When they first met, he was the perfect gentleman, a complete charmer. At dinner parties he was the life and soul of the group. Her best friend thought he was terrific. Her mother thought he was the great provider. Everyone thought she was so lucky.

But after they were married, she began to see a different side of him. Gradually he managed to cut her off from her friends – though at the time she hardly noticed what was happening. He began to turn down invitations to dinner parties they had once enjoyed. Sometimes, if they did see other people, he would very subtly put her down, laugh at her opinions or make her feel like a fool in front of them, often in ways only she understood, leaving her feeling uncomfortable.

Afterwards, if she was upset, he would put his arm around her and say things like: 'You know I was only teasing, darling. Don't take it so personally.' Then he would be attentive and considerate again, and enthusiastic about their life together. He would tell her that they could not live without each other, that he needed her and that nobody else had what they had. If she talked to friends about her niggles over his behaviour, they could not understand what was worrying her. As far as they could see he was a kind, caring man. Everyone has their problems, they agreed, but that was all there was to it.

For long periods everything would be 'normal' and peaceful but then he would do or say something which would completely throw her. When she decided to do something for herself, for example to take up some part-time studying at home, he was so outraged that he burnt her lifetime's collection of diaries, drawings and books in the fire.

When she was in hospital having their first child, she waited every day for him to visit, but he never came. Then, when she brought the baby home, she opened the living-room door to find the word 'slut' traced in the thin layer of dust on the coffee table which had accumulated while she was away. Mortified as she was, she bit her tongue, because she wanted them to be happy with the new baby.

His moods became more unpredictable. If his dinner was not on the table when he came home, or she was talking to a friend on the telephone, he could be angry and abusive, or cold and distant. He made all the decisions, and expected her to accept them without question. When she stood up for herself, and tried to develop outside interests, he even threatened to have her committed to a psychiatric hospital. There must be something wrong with her, he argued, if she was not happy looking after him and her children. Why did she need anything else?

Their friends were like his echoes. They could not see why she seemed discontented. Unwittingly they made her feel that it must be her fault if she was not happy. She got tired of people starting sentences with 'But he's so nice', implying that she was some sort of dragon, that she was on edge, snappy and irritable.

This woman is not alone. Having worked with abused women since 1979, I know that her misery is shared by thousands of women, who may have no cuts, bruises or scars but who only know that they are miserable in their relationships. Many women are immobilised by the effects of years and years of subtle, all-pervading emotional and verbal abuse, without ever thinking of themselves as abused at all. Surely that is something which happens to other people?

Many of these women seem to be strong, confident, capable people. Some are qualified professional women, who appear to have perfect marriages and relationships. No one knows that deep down they feel unfulfilled and dissatisfied, not knowing why the control they exercise over their job is lacking in their relationship with their partner. With him they continually mind their Ps and Qs and alter their behaviour to make life more tolerable. They are unable to be themselves.

Yet should anyone suggest that they are abused, they would say, 'Don't be silly.' Even if there are things that disturb them, they frequently gloss over them, make excuses for their partner's behaviour, or convince themselves that they are imagining things, often because they cannot bear to admit either to themselves or to colleagues and friends that their relationship is less than wonderful. After all, they are married to the most charming man in the world. If they complain to friends who see their partner only as a nice friendly guy, they run the risk of appearing to do nothing but put their husband or boyfriend down. Often the result is that the man ends up with all the sympathy.

Often, too, the incidents which worry them seem so trivial when taken on their own. Many women who ring Refuge begin by apologising for asking for help over something which they think sounds silly. They do not believe they have the right to ask for assistance when they have no physical wounds to show for their distress. One woman rang me, saying, 'I shouldn't really be calling you. I'm probably wasting your time. I'm not really one of your women. He doesn't hit me, but I know there's something wrong with our relationship...'

What many women are unaware of, since they do not even realise that they are being abused, is that their desperation and confusion, their lack of autonomy, is a direct result of their partner's abusive behaviour.

Do not think for a moment that I am dismissing the thousands of women who come to Refuge with hideous wounds, women who are literally scared for their lives. But the vast majority of the women who come to us for help are subjected to relentless controlling and demeaning behaviour, whether or not physical abuse is involved.

Headline news only highlights the more sensational stories – but scalded limbs, broken bones, wounds from knives and hatchets, and murder threats are not the only legacies of the abuser. Emotional and mental abuse leaves scars as deep as physical wounds. And many women live with such abuse as *well* as physical beatings.

Many of the women I talk to in my work are so continually degraded, demoralised and humiliated by their partners that they have lost all confidence in themselves. They feel constantly undermined. They are despairing and confused. What is more, they feel terribly alone. Because they have no bruises to show, they think no one will understand.

Today, law-makers and the public have begun to understand that domestic violence is about more than black eyes and broken bones. Some of the different techniques an abuser may use to control his partner are now recognised in law, thanks to the government's new legislation around coercive control, which came into effect in 2015. Since I wrote the first edition of this book, there has been a shift in public attitudes when it comes to domestic violence. Now, domestic violence appears on the front pages of newspapers and in the nation's favourite soap operas. Thanks to this increased awareness, many more women now know there is support and they do not need to suffer in silence. Legislation has been strengthened, showing women – and the men who abuse them – that domestic violence is a crime and is unacceptable.

Yet domestic violence is still the biggest issue affecting women and children in our society. *Still*, one in four women experiences it.[1] *Still*, two women are killed by their current or former partner every single week in England and Wales alone.[2] The National Domestic Violence Helpline, which Refuge runs with Women's Aid, receives almost 87,000 calls a year, often from women fearing for their lives. Twenty-five years on from the first edition of this book, the scale of woman abuse in the UK remains depressingly high. And these are just the women who seek support – what about those who continue to suffer in silence?

Back then, I wanted to know why so many women are abused – both physically and emotionally. I wanted to know why men think they have the right to behave in such a controlling, domineering way towards their partners. I talked to hundreds of women, and delved into reams of research on abused women and the men who abuse them. The book became my attempt to explain why men abuse women and at the same time to provide hope for the future.

Since then the number of women Refuge supports on any given day has grown year on year. I have met women from all walks of life, from all nationalities and cultures, who have experienced many forms of woman abuse – often simultaneously. A woman who is being abused by her partner may also have been forced into prostitution by him or forced to marry him against her will. Many women face additional barriers to safety beyond their gender: racism is still prevalent in this country and as austerity bites, it is the services for black, Asian, minority ethnic and refugee women that tend to close first. However, I am more convinced than ever that the root cause of all woman abuse – from rape and sexual assault, to so-called 'honour'-based violence, to female genital mutilation, to modern slavery – is the same: men exerting power over women.

In the first edition, I shared my belief that the predominant reason why men behave in this way is because we live in a society which, frankly, allows – indeed encourages – them to do so; a society which bombards us with messages that men are dominant and powerful, and that women are nothing without them, that women are dependent on men for their sense of self-worth and security; a society which makes it hard for women who want to leave their abusers to find houses, jobs, childcare and so on; a society which implies that women bring abuse on themselves. 'She must have provoked it,' people say.

I should add that in stressing the role of society, I am not dismissing individual psychological factors in woman abuse; but they are factors, not causes. My concern was – and is – to show that woman abuse is a *pattern* of behaviour. Men who abuse behave in remarkably similar ways, as indeed do women who are abused. We can learn to recognise this pattern, and in doing so we will see how it is the product of social conditioning.

Twenty-five years on from the first edition, the fundamental message of this book remains the same. The pattern of men controlling women endures. It endures because sexism continues to permeate almost every aspect of women's public and private lives, as I will discuss in Chapter 5. What has evolved, though, are some of the *methods* of control. Who could have predicted then, the extent to which technology and the internet would affect the life of the abused woman? Now the abusive man has an array of new weapons in his armoury, which – should he so wish – allow him to terrorise and control a woman from a distance, or without ever even meeting her. More often than not, though, technology is used in tandem with other techniques of control. Now in Refuge's services, the majority of women have experienced abuse through technology, from receiving abusive text messages or emails to having a tracker placed on their car.

As Emmeline Pankhurst observed, 'As a river cannot flow higher than its source, so a society cannot be judged higher than the way it treats its women.' Well, despite the great strides that women have made since Emmeline Pankhurst made her stand, women are still devalued and discriminated against. And if we go on implying that women are not that important, it is inevitable that many men will take the same attitude in their individual relationships. And the consequence, frequently, is woman abuse.

Of course, not all men abuse women. Some men reject society's messages, and their relationships are based on equality and respect. Yet there are still a frightening number of men who are unable to behave like that. I want to show women that they are not alone, that what they are going through is part of a much wider scenario.

I am writing this second edition not only to share new insights from my work at Refuge, but because the root causes of violence against women – sexism and gender inequality – remain stubbornly prevalent. I am writing in the hope that our society might acknowledge – and ultimately change – some of the subtle ways in which we give men permission to abuse women. Above all, I am writing this to let abused women know that, whether they stay or leave, they have choices. Women can escape the tyranny of abuse and begin to unravel their feelings and rebuild their lives. Chapter 6 deals with the emotions – including grief and loss – abused women may encounter as they come to recognise that they cannot change their partner's behaviour. I am writing in the hope that women may feel more empowered and better equipped to reclaim their lives.

Because I talk to abused women almost every day of my life, I am using their stories to highlight the behaviour of their partners. But – despite the fact that the immediate concern of Refuge is to provide women with safety and support – my overriding concern is to shift the spotlight from the women onto the men, and onto our society as a whole. A society which says, 'But he can't be abusive. He's so charming.'

# CHAPTER 1

# Charm Syndrome Man

'The Charm Syndrome' is a distinct pattern of behaviour. It is a man's use of charm to gain control over a woman. Once he has achieved that control, Charm Syndrome Man may or may not continue to charm his partner. But what he will always do is assert and reinforce his control by emotional and sometimes physical abuse.

When Melinda met Trevor, she was 'devastated' by his charm. 'He was very good-looking, highly intelligent. Very, very charming. I liked him a lot, we were very good companions, and he was fun to be with,' she told me. Eleven months later, after Melinda and Trevor had married and had had their first baby, he hit her for the first time. It was the beginning of a 12-year nightmare which ended only in divorce.

Melinda is 32, outgoing, bright, with a demanding and well-paid job in the city. Trevor is highly intelligent, a man who regretted not going to university after he left school. When he and Melinda met, she was more than happy to support him, so that he could become a mature student.

Melinda hardly fits the picture most people have of an abused woman as a careworn, pathetic creature, suffering at the hands of a husband who has one too many at the pub, then comes home and beats her in a drunken rage. Trevor only drank socially, and was the kind of guy that everyone liked. He was fun, good-looking, an entertaining conversationalist. 'He actually *liked* me, quite separately from everything else,' she says. 'He put me on a pedestal really. No one was allowed to swear in front of me, and as far as he was concerned, I was a real lady. He'd do all sorts of things for me – he used to hitchhike to London to see me and things like that.

He made me feel special, unique really. He said that no other woman had made him feel so good, so loved. We were going to make a great team. He needed me, it was the two of us against the world.'

The men who abuse women may be refuse collectors, accountants, bus drivers or film producers. I have counselled women who have suffered terribly at the hands of policemen, clergymen and judges. When I worked in the refuge I was horrified to find myself counselling the wife of a lawyer who supported our work and was at that very time actually involved in proceedings on behalf of an abused wife, before going home to hit his own.

What these men have in common is that they are invariably the last people anyone would suspect of abusing their partners. They are the 'nice guys from next door' who are always willing to do a neighbour a favour: they will mend the plumbing, weed the garden, jump-start the car. They may be the men who seem to uphold strict moral standards, who are popular at parties or in the local pub. Or they may be quiet, 'steady' chaps, the ones 'you can always rely on'. Charm Syndrome Men present a likeable face to the rest of the world: charm obscures the abuser. And being liked feeds their self-image.

Some are intensely charismatic. During 1988–1989 the whole of America watched the trial of criminal lawyer Joel Steinberg, who had physically abused his lover, Hedda Nussbaum, so badly (on top of years of emotional abuse) that according to *Newsweek* magazine her face was distorted like 'a boxer's'. He was also charged with the murder of their adopted daughter. Over a six-year period he broke Hedda Nussbaum's knee and some ribs, choked her hard enough to damage her vocal cords, burned her body with a propane torch, knocked out her teeth, pulled out her hair, poked his fingers in her eyes and urinated on her.

In a court transcript, she told how she fell in love with Steinberg. 'I loved to listen to him,' she said. 'Basically, I worshipped him. He was the most wonderful man I had ever met. I believed he had supernatural, godlike power. He would praise me and build my ego.

On the other hand, he was constantly critical. And he would strike me.' As we will see, Joel's manipulation typifies the way many men in this book behave – alternating charm with abuse.

During the same decade, the Charlotte Fedders case also hit the headlines, after her husband John – another lawyer – had admitted in court to having beaten his wife on several occasions during their 18-year marriage. The judge in the Fedders case said: 'When you put it all together, you have as classic a situation of cruelty...and a classic situation of excessively vicious conduct...as one can find.'[3] John Fedders was the man about whom she had said when they first met, 'I knew he was the one love of my life.' In Fedders' book *Shattered Dreams* her co-author, Laura Elliott, talks of how Charlotte could hardly believe her luck that she had made such a catch. John, she says, was charming and witty – so romantic that he took her to see *The Sound of Music* and held her hand during the wedding scene.[4] But before long the beatings began. The irony is that he eventually won 25 per cent of the royalties from *Shattered Dreams*.[5]

The men who abuse women may be glamorous and famous and there are countless examples of well-known actors, pop stars and sportsmen who have admitted in court and elsewhere to physical abuse of their partners. One only has to think of Ulrika Jonsson, Sheryl Gascoigne and Rihanna, or read Tina Turner's book *I, Tina*, for examples of how an apparently glamorous and exciting life can be a personal secret nightmare. The late actress Lynda Bellingham also spoke about the repeated threats she received from her second husband. She successfully brought him to court, after which he was banned from contacting her or going near her home for seven years.

What is especially notable is that, whether their husbands are movie stars or lawyers or accounts clerks, in more or less the same breath as they describe their humiliation and pain, most abused women talk of the loving, caring, *charming* side of the men who abuse them. 'He could charm the birds out of the trees' is a phrase

I hear over and over again. These women invariably remember the charming side of their partners, the side they fell in love with. They describe them as loving, tender, funny and considerate. More often than not, they explain that in between bouts of abuse their partners revert to being charmers. They can beg forgiveness, smother them in affection and promise they will never behave badly again. And because the women still care, they agree to give it just one more try…

That word charm has cropped up again and again. At first it seemed astonishing, but soon – and repeatedly – I was making the connection between these two apparent opposites, charm and abuse, which seemed to run like two threads intertwined in the tapestry of these women's lives. It might be the charm of Dr Jekyll and the abuse of Mr Hyde – and, just as in Stevenson's novel, the activities of Mr Hyde are protected by the character of Dr Jekyll.

This is what I have come to call the Charm Syndrome.

Melinda is one of six women whose stories I have chosen to tell – because they are so typical. Let me introduce the others (naturally names and other details have been changed, to protect the identities of those involved).

Beverley is a 28-year-old fashion model, a stylish, attractive young woman who loves her work. The first time she met Dave, a singer who was performing in a nightclub, she remembers that 'He was totally charming, terribly well dressed, the perfect gentleman. He stood up on the stage and sang love songs looking into my eyes, and I fell for it. He seemed so together, very confident, but soft behind, very loving, very romantic. He'd take me out to dinner and let everyone know how he felt about me. He made me feel special.

'During the first six months we couldn't get enough of each other. No expense was spared. If we went on a picnic, he would have picked the most romantic spot, miles from anywhere, overlooking the sea. When we were mellow with vintage wine he would read me love poems. I couldn't believe my luck. He was so attentive. I never had to worry about a thing.

'I was in awe of him. He seemed such an amazing person. He knew about everything. He would always help me if there was anything I couldn't manage on my own. Our sex life was fantastic. He made everything seem so exciting – even doing the shopping. In the supermarket queue he would whisper that he wanted to make love to me the moment we got back.'

Hazel is a 24-year-old hairdresser. Her husband Jimmy is a builder. They met at a party. 'He could make you feel as though you were the only woman who had ever existed, he was so charming,' says Hazel. 'He would take me for long walks, and hold my hand. He was so attentive, as if his whole world was wrapped up in you. He could really charm the birds out of the trees.

'He had these great ideas, dreams really, about how he was going to build my ideal house for me. He'd sit for hours telling me the way he'd decorate it, where it would be, what the garden would be like . . . it all sounded so wonderful. It made me feel really important – he was going to do all these things just for me. I'd always wanted a lovely house and someone like Jimmy, so it was a bit like a dream come true.'

Rebecca was 46 when she met Ralph, a solicitor. She had been widowed for several years and had three small children. Everyone thought of Ralph as a fine, upstanding man. He was ten years older than her, and had been married before, but he had been divorced for many years. He and Rebecca were introduced at a dinner party, discovered they shared a love of music and the theatre, and began to see each other regularly.

'When I thought of other men I had been out with,' says Rebecca, 'Ralph seemed perfect. Our mutual love of music brought us close together. We sang in a local choral society, which was a wonderful experience. We both loved walking, golf and tennis. He was very gentle and seemed to be fun-loving, on the spur of the moment suggesting outings to cafés, art galleries or concerts. He was extremely protective of me. He was very conscientious about his work as a solicitor and concerned about moral issues. I was impressed by that. He had such a strong sense of justice. He seemed so competent – you know, able to manage everything, yet at the same time so calm. I had never come across someone who provided such a sense of solidity. My friends, too, were won over by him. They thought he had real charm and told me how lucky I was.'

When Sally met Guy, she was a student at a polytechnic where he was a lecturer. 'I think I was bewitched by him,' she recalls. 'He was a very magnetic, educated, articulate man. I was studying for my finals, and he kept saying I'd work better if I took more time off to relax. He said, "Trust me. I'll look after you." And that is what I did, I suppose – trust him, I mean. And I did pass my finals. I can't think how, considering how much time I spent with him. He sort of took me over. We got completely wrapped up in each other. Before my exams he sent a message saying, "Good luck. I love you." He was wonderfully charming and I was flattered.'

Everyone thought that Laura and James had the perfect teenage romance. They met when he was at a public school and she was at an expensive girls' school. Both went to university but their relationship endured and when Laura was 25 they were married. 'He was a bright, witty, amusing person to be with,' says Laura. 'He was very attractive physically, everyone thought he was charming. We seemed to have a terrific relationship. I thought we were very lucky.'

I have met countless women either socially or in the course of my work, whose stories are astonishingly similar to those of these six women. The details and extent of abuse are different, yet invariably when I ask these women, 'What was he like when you first met?' the answer is the same. Each of these men, in his own way, is a charmer. Not just in the eyes of their partners, but in the eyes of many people they meet. Not only do they charm their partners, but they are able to get away with behaving abusively because unconsciously they use charm to convince everyone (including themselves) that they are great guys. After all, how could such terrific characters be abusers? This is vital to their self-image, which requires that they deny that they are abusers.

They may not all be witty, magnetic men, who can be extravagant in their affection. They may not all give red roses, buy champagne and quote Shakespeare. They may be 'rough diamonds': unsophisticated and inarticulate, or they may be quiet, undemonstrative types whose charm lies in their apparent solidity and dependability. But the common characteristic all these men share is their ability to make a woman feel special. To charm them. Many abusers, in fact, are womanisers.

The *Concise Oxford English Dictionary* defines the verb 'to charm' as 'use one's charm in order to influence (someone)' and 'control or achieve by or as if by magic'. This is something completely different from being 'a nice guy', someone who is simply amusing and fun. Charm is, in fact, manipulative. To use charm is to influence, to bewitch someone, to bring them within your power. Ultimately to control them.

And that is the key word: *control.*

Of course it is possible for a man to be charming, to bewitch women, yet not to abuse them. The self-gratification he enjoys when a woman is besotted with him is often enough. But in the case of Charm Syndrome Man, he uses his charm to the ultimate, because it is *control* over his partner that he really wants. And he uses his charm to deceive others too.

My definition of woman abuse is this: systematic, patterned behaviour on the part of the abusive man, designed – consciously or subconsciously – to control and dominate 'his woman'. And in the armoury of the abuser, charm is both an essential weapon and a disguise...

# CHAPTER 2

# A Pattern of Control

The first cracks in the charmer's make-up often begin to show once a woman has committed herself to him. One woman I helped told me that the violence began on her wedding night, when the man she had thought was 'so gorgeous, somebody to love me', slapped her for the first time.

Sally recalls the first time she was shocked by Guy's behaviour. 'We had been going to go out together on a Saturday, and he had to cancel it because he'd had to do an extra tutorial. After he'd gone, I was a bit bored so I rang up some girlfriends and we went bathing in the river. When Guy came home I told him, and he was furious that I had spent the day enjoying myself without him. He hardly spoke to me for days. I couldn't understand it. He had never behaved like that before and it threw me completely.'

The only time Laura recalls being confused at James's behaviour when they first started going out together was when she had gone to see a new play with some girlfriends, on a night when he was playing rugby. 'When he came home, I thought he'd be really interested to hear about the play,' she says, 'but instead he was really hurt that I had gone without him. He kept saying that that was the sort of special thing we should do together – and why hadn't I asked him to go. I had only gone on that night because I usually sat in while he played rugby. I felt so guilty at not putting him first, that I never did it again. Crazy, isn't it?'

It may be days, months or years before an abuser begins to wound his partner with blows or words, but whenever it begins it is devastating for the woman. What has happened to Mr Right? Where is the charmer, the man who can make a woman feel so loved, and appreciated, and special? And when the abuse begins after years, it is likely that it really began long before and that the woman simply failed to identify it.

Charm Syndrome Man begins to abuse when he feels he can take his partner for granted. Once he has persuaded the woman that he is the ideal man she has been searching for all her life, once she has committed herself to marriage or to a permanent relationship, Charm Syndrome Man no longer feels the need to charm her. He has used charm to control her for so long that she has become used to responding to his suggestions. Now he needs to charm her only in the moments when he fears he may be losing his control over her; for control is what a relationship is all about, as far as Charm Syndrome Man is concerned.

In my experience, women rarely have any way of knowing that they are embarking on life with an abusive man. By the time they find out, they are so embroiled in the relationship that it is very difficult to walk away. Looking back, some women recall 'niggles' early on in the relationship: perhaps an uncalled-for bout of jealousy, a temper tantrum or an unexpected verbal attack, but usually they dismiss it once their partner's good side reappears. Warning signals are written off as isolated incidents, because Charm Syndrome Man has an extraordinary ability to manipulate people, to cloak the controlling side of his nature with charm. As Sally explains: 'I think that I was rather dazed by the sudden changes in Guy's behaviour, but because things went back to normal pretty quickly, and he would be loving and considerate until the next incident, I didn't let it bother me too much.'

An abusive man may use a whole range of weapons to control his partner, from actual physical abuse to verbal, emotional, psychological, sexual, financial or social abuse. Remember, non-physical forms of abuse are as potent in destroying a woman's confidence and personality as violence, though they may be less obvious. An abuser can cripple his partner emotionally by humiliating and degrading her, just as surely as he can wound her with blows.

And always, just when he senses that she may be on the point of walking out, Charm Syndrome Man resorts to his greatest weapon: charm. He may say he is sorry, tell her he loves her, that he hates himself for acting the way he did, it was only because he was under stress, or had had too much to drink, that it will never happen again... that he needs her support more than ever. 'After all we've been through, how can you throw away the most important relationship you've ever had?' is a typical plea. Charm Syndrome Man uses charm to confuse his partner, to make her forget the bad times and bind her to him further. As one woman, looking back on her relationship, described it: 'It's like being a fish on a hook.'

Like Sally, the majority of the women Refuge supports only recognise their perpetrator's pattern of abuse after they have escaped it. It is sometimes easier for a woman to dismiss abusive incidents as one-offs – 'He was just having a bad day, he had drunk too much,' she might say. This is understandable; how can we expect a woman to recognise the pattern of abuse in her own relationship when society as a whole refuses to see male violence for what it is?

Take domestic fatalities. In England and Wales, two women are killed by their partner or former partner every single week. To put this figure in context: during the UK's involvement in military action in Afghanistan (2001–2014), 453 members of the British Armed Forces lost their lives. In that same period, more than 1,000 women were killed in the context of domestic violence. In addition, an estimated three women commit suicide per week because of domestic violence.[6] Then there are the women killed by their sons, brothers or fathers – and the women killed outside of a domestic setting, by strange men or by men they barely know. There is little official data on the extent of the problem, but Refuge's 'Know Her Name' campaign revealed that in just three years (between 2010 and 2013), 268 women were killed in the context of domestic violence. What if elderly people were being slaughtered in their homes at such an alarming rate? Or people of a particular faith? Society and the media would assume they were part of a pattern. Newspaper columnists would rightly hand-wring about hate crime and demand action from politicians. But not when it comes to women. These are not a series of unrelated deaths; they are women being killed *because* they are women.

An abuser killing 'his woman' is the ultimate manifestation of his need to control her and prevent her from leaving. Women are at the greatest risk of homicide at the point of separation or after leaving a violent partner.[7] When the abuser realises he is losing his grip, he may resort to extreme measures. Of course, long before this final act is played out, the abuser has slowly, purposefully, built up his pattern of control – a pattern that begins with charm.

In the following sections I shall look at the ways in which Charm Syndrome Man controls his partner. There is no definitive checklist of abuse, nothing to say that a man is necessarily abusive because he is possessive, jealous, tight with money or prefers his wife to stay at home rather than work. A woman needs to look at every area of her relationship and see if there is a pattern. Ultimately, she needs to ask herself whether or not she is in control of her own life, or whether it is her partner who pulls the strings.

If a woman is afraid to be herself or avoids doing certain things because she is afraid of her partner's reaction, if he prevents her from acting the way she wants to or makes her do things against her will by using physical force, verbal abuse, threats or bullying, or if he confuses her by treating her contemptuously one moment and lovingly the next, then she is being abused. And all the more so if she *feels* she is being abused.


## 'He always had to be the boss'

'We were playing a game of Monopoly,' says Beverley, the fashion model, 'and in the middle of the game, Dave stood up, tipped the board upside down and accused me of cheating, then he stormed out of the place. And I said, "My God, it's only a game." But as the relationship went on, it was as if he had to win at everything – that was really important. He had to prove to himself all the time that he was better than me and he took great delight in putting me down in front of everyone.'

In his bid for control, an abusive man tries to dominate every aspect of his partner's life. He may phone or text message constantly – whether his partner is at home or work – to check up on what she is doing, using the flimsiest of excuses, such as 'Can you buy a roll of Sellotape for my desk?' or 'Don't forget to pick up the dry cleaning.' He constantly has to prove he is boss even over the tiniest details, such as the clothes his partner wears, or which TV programmes to watch. In one headline-hitting case a man actually killed his wife for putting the mustard pot in the 'wrong' place on the table.

After Rebecca and Ralph, the solicitor, were married, she began to notice that he made more and more of the decisions. She told me: 'If I was really interested in watching a nature documentary, he would insist on watching a crime drama. I knew it was useless to express any interest in a programme. Then when *he* had had enough TV for the evening, he would go over and switch off, then rip the plug out of the wall, leave the room and turn off the light, leaving me in darkness, as though I didn't even exist. But if I wanted to go to bed early and read a book, there was no question of it. I had to sit up and watch the late news with him.

'When I was on the phone, he would come along and shout, "Goodbye!" to make me hang up. Then if I still carried on the conversation, he would just come over and press the button to cut me off, gloating while he did it.

'I know it all sounds so unimportant, but it built up to be so incredibly oppressive. Once he drove me so mad I went out into the night – it was in the middle of winter and it was snowing, but I was furious and I couldn't care less. I just wanted to get out of that oppressive atmosphere.

'I could never suggest we go out. It always had to be his idea. And if we did go anywhere and I was frantically trying to get the children dressed, Ralph would go out and sit in the car and hoot the horn aggressively to hurry me up. If for some reason he had forgotten something and had to go back into the house, that was a different matter.'

An abusive man often has clear rules about the space in the house – if there is a spare room he will commandeer it for his study, in which he cannot be disturbed. His possessions must not be moved or touched by anyone.

Ralph had his own bathroom. 'Nobody else was allowed in it,' Rebecca says. 'His excuse was that he had to get to work on time, but he still didn't allow anyone to use it at the weekends. He was absolutely obsessive about everything. Everything had to be in the right place. The children's toys had to be put away before he came home.'

Ralph made his point about who was boss in petty ways. On one occasion when she had just cooked dinner, Rebecca says, 'I was walking from the kitchen to the table with a heavy casserole, to put it on the table, and Ralph was standing in my way. Now, I am sure if you did this and your husband was standing there he would move without a word, but Ralph didn't move out of the way and I was nearly dropping the casserole. It was red hot. I said, "Come on, Ralph, let me put it down," and he said, "Walk around me." And from then on his attitude was "*I am me* and you must not encroach on my territory."'

Guy insisted that Sally keep her books upstairs, while *his* should be on display downstairs. 'His books were more important, more intellectual. And there were so many other things,' says Sally. 'For instance, he had his desk in the living room, where the television and stereo were, but I felt I couldn't go in there while he was working. I couldn't play his vinyl records, because I'd scratch them, and I couldn't play mine because he said they weren't in good enough condition and they would damage his stylus. When I was watching television with a friend once, he came in and started to chip the paint off a metal cupboard he wanted to repaint. It made screeching noises, like fingernails on a blackboard, but at first I tried to ignore it, rather than start a row. When it was really driving me crazy, and I asked him to stop, he just gave me a long hard stare – he had these really penetrating dark-brown eyes – and carried on chipping.

'There was no escaping him even when he was away. He expected me to come home straight away after work to let his dog out, and after that it wasn't worth driving all the way back into town. I realise now that I hadn't got a life of my own. Even when he was out of the house I felt him as a heavy presence.'

An abuser has rigid ideas about the roles of men and women: men make the rules, and women obey them. Women, he believes, are emotional and incapable of rational thought – unlike men. That men are rational, women intuitive, is a distinction taught by a male-dominated society: irrational, emotional women cannot be trusted with decision-taking. Their role is in the background. So, in an abuser's view, the very fact of being a man gives him certain privileges. He believes that the woman's place is to stay at home with the children, so that *he* can go out. Jimmy the builder was a case in point. After he and Hazel were married there were no more romantic walks in the park. 'He was more interested in his mates than in me,' she says. Soon after the wedding she became pregnant and, once the baby was born, he was out more than ever. 'He would never ever say: "I must get home to Hazel and the baby." He would say, "I'm the master of the house. If I want to stay out all night long drinking, I can." He had to be the master, he had to be the boss and he had to let everybody else know it.

'He was always going out, and on one occasion I thought, "It's my turn," so I asked him if I could go, and he said okay. When I was about to leave, he knocked me all around the kitchen, saying, "Where do you think you're going then?" He insisted that I had to stay in because *he'd* made arrangements with a friend – I later discovered the "friend" was a barmaid in the pub around the corner, and everyone knew what was going on, apart from me.

'I was so frightened, I ran round to my mother's house for help, but she's a really strong Catholic, and her attitude is that marriage is sacred, and you have to work at it. She kept telling me that I had to be forgiving and try harder to make it work. She said that her life hadn't been a bed of roses either, and that women can't expect to have perfect marriages. I think if I'd had somebody to encourage me at that point, I would have packed my bags and left, but the very person I thought would support me was saying, "Go back and try harder." It just made me feel even more alone.'

Often the incidents over which Charm Syndrome Man makes such a fuss seem quite trivial, and it is invariably easier for a woman to go along with her partner's wishes, just to keep the peace – but after a while this constant interference in her life, and the strain of forever trying to anticipate his needs in order to prevent physical or verbal abuse, can become oppressive and debilitating.

Guy made Sally's life hell by trying to dominate the decision-making. She says, 'I can remember one time when we were deciding how to decorate our first flat. We had a row about what colour to do it in and he got really angry. It wasn't a case of just having a difference of opinion over colours – I was expecting that – but he just started screaming, "You stupid bitch!" I was shocked and hurt. He made me feel so small. But I thought it wasn't worth the aggravation, so I gave in and painted the wall a bright red – horrible!' she laughs. 'He didn't help at all. He only seemed interested in winning the battle.

'I can think of something else, although to an outsider it might seem trivial, but in actual fact he was being unreasonable. I used to love cooking fantastic meals and he used to love eating them. He actively encouraged me and bragged about my culinary skills to his friends. So of course I went out of my way to please him even more, spending my grant money on expensive ingredients. Then suddenly he would accusingly tell me that he had put on weight because of my cooking...so I would prepare less fattening food for a while only to be criticised for not bothering. I couldn't win.

'I was willing to put up with his idiosyncrasies partly because I thought that is the price you pay for living with a genius, and also because I was sure that every relationship had its ups and downs.

After all, most of the time he was wonderfully charming and romantic and everyone liked him.'

Guy changed so easily from charmer to boor that Sally was constantly 'walking on eggshells', never sure when the tiniest thing would spark off a torrent of abuse. 'Over time,' she says, 'his behaviour became more and more unpredictable. I never knew what would upset him next.

'In the beginning he had encouraged me to talk about my work. But after we'd been living together for a while, if I started to discuss it with him, he would tap his watch after only a few moments, sigh, turn eyes to the ceiling and tell me my time was up. At other times he would seem genuinely interested and encourage me to talk, and then after some time he would stop me dead and say I had gone over the time limit. It was so humiliating and infuriating, but I never challenged him.

'He was very precise about time. He used to get really upset if I was late, even a few minutes. Once I had invited a girlfriend I hadn't seen for years to stop by and have tea, and also meet Guy for the first time. I thought I would stop off at the bakery on my way home to buy something nice for the occasion.

'I was *six* minutes late. When I said hello Guy just glared at me. I couldn't imagine what I had done wrong. He was angry that I was late – a whole six minutes – and demanded a detailed account of where I had been during the six minutes. When my girlfriend arrived he went into the bedroom and refused to come out. She thought it was all very strange, especially as she had come over partly to meet him. I was so embarrassed, but even those feelings had to be suppressed. Later he spent hours telling me that he wouldn't have behaved that way if I hadn't been late. In the end I felt responsible for the whole thing and wound up apologising to *him*!'

Guy, in true Charm Syndrome fashion, could never accept that he was less than perfect. Nothing could be wrong with *his* behaviour – Sally must have forced him to act that way. It takes time to realise just how easily an abusive man can manipulate his partner into believing that everything is *her* fault, not *his*. Similarly, it takes time to realise that the relationship is abusive. Some women think the abuse is just a passing phase – after all, as Sally remarked, every relationship has its ups and downs.

Hazel's husband Jimmy also had to have his way over every little detail. She told me: 'He had to have everything just right. I never had time to think what I wanted. I always had to do everything to make him happy, like keeping the baby quiet. If we went out, I had to look happy or I'd get a hiding when I got home. People might have thought I *was* happy, but he was pulling the strings. If it was a toss-up between using money to buy food or him going for a drink, it had to go on drink. If I disagreed with something – anything he wanted and I wouldn't go along with – I got a hiding.'

Abusive men are frequently fanatical about the most trivial things. 'Guy was always very precise,' says Sally. 'Our spontaneous, exotic gourmet dinners turned into a kind of competition. Romantic moments were spoiled when he would measure our wine glasses to make sure I didn't have more than him. Towards the end of the relationship I used to practically fill his glass right up to the edge. As soon as he had a sip I would fill his glass up again.'

When Rebecca first met Ralph, she was impressed by the fact that 'he seemed so competent – you know, able to manage everything. He was extremely reliable.' When he phoned her every day to say what time he would arrive home from the office, she took it as a sign of his consideration. She soon realised that it was his way of signalling what time he wanted his dinner on the table – and if it wasn't ready, he would create an atmosphere for the rest of the evening. It was also a ploy on his behalf to make sure she stayed home in the evenings, to wait for his call.

'When we first lived in the country we had just one car and I used to drive Ralph the 12 miles to the station and then drive home again,' says Rebecca. 'I had to wait for him to call from the office every night between 5.40 and 7.15. He would tell me which train he would catch, what time it left Victoria and what time it would arrive at our local station. This meant that if anyone else phoned up during the time he wanted to call, I would have to be quite short with them, because Ralph would be furious if he rang up and the line was engaged.

'I felt I had to comply with his demands because I didn't work (no wife of his was going to work for a living!), therefore he held the purse strings and the least I could do was ferry him back and forth to the station, so he could bring home the money.

'Even when we had two cars I was amazed to find that he still insisted on this arrangement rather than leaving one of the cars at the station all day. I can see now that it was part of the control scenario. At the time I was willing to go along with it – I was a complete puppet – but I did find it all an enormous strain, especially with three lively children to care for. After a day of freedom from his rigid rules we suddenly all had to rush around putting everything back in exactly the right place and making out that nothing had moved all day long.

'Strangely enough I grew to appreciate his phone calls as warning signals. They gave us time to psych ourselves up for his homecoming.'

Laughingly Rebecca admits, 'One of the things which irritated me most was that he would never let me sit on the edge of the sofa. He said it ruined it – so I used to take great delight in walking all over the sofa when he was out! Just for the hell of it!'

## 'He was jealous of everything and everybody'

Like many women who believe they have found the perfect partner, Beverley was shocked the first time Dave flew into a jealous rage, but she dismissed it as an isolated incident. 'It was only three months after we got together. Our relationship couldn't have been better, and by that time he'd asked me to marry him,' she recalls. 'We were at his family home. His parents had gone away on holiday and I was just wearing a dressing-gown of his. Some man was mentioned, I can't remember what was said, but I just remember that he spat at me, spat at my face, and then pushed me against a wall, which ripped this dressing-gown – which I came to realise later was absolutely nothing! I was hysterical. I was absolutely frightened to death and ran out of the house.

'I couldn't believe it, I was going to marry this man, and I couldn't believe it wasn't going to work. I thought it was just an outburst. I didn't realise there would be more and worse. Apparently I slept with everybody – which I didn't do, and wouldn't do either, because I'm a very monogamous person, a fact which Dave would never believe.'

The very possibility, however imaginary, that his partner might be unfaithful to him assumes enormous proportions in the mind of Charm Syndrome Man, because it undermines his control over her. Not only that, but he risks being ridiculed by the outside world as 'less than a real man' because he cannot keep his own wife in line. Her past boyfriends, current friends, the children, even inanimate objects she treasures, appear to him as threats. He is jealous of her job, particularly if she is more successful than he is, and suspicious of her colleagues. He may try to entice her to work in the same place as him, suggesting that he hates to be apart from her, or it is another area of their life they can share. His real motive is that he wants to keep an eye on her.

An abuser's fears are almost always totally unfounded. Melinda told me: 'I am the most faithful person in the world, I couldn't have been more faithful – it is anathema to me to have affairs or anything like that. And I never looked at anybody else, it just didn't occur to me, and somewhere he knew that.'

However, many abusers constantly imagine that their partners have lovers, becoming so suspicious that they subject them to hours of interrogation and accusation. Ironically, for most abused women, cheating on a partner is the last thing on their minds. Many women are either too frightened of the consequences of being found out, or they have come to think that all men are abusive, so why would they jump out of the frying pan into the fire? Even so, women often tell me that they end up confessing to things they haven't done, just to be left alone. They may be beaten as a result, but at least the harassment stops for a while.

An abuser also uses jealousy as a weapon to isolate his partner: if seeing friends and family (of either sex), keeping in touch with previous boyfriends and husbands, or even talking to other men causes him to create such a storm of physical or verbal abuse, it is easier for the woman to avoid outside contact. Once again, she is changing and moulding her behaviour in an attempt to keep the peace. And because his jealousy isolates her, she becomes more dependent on him to answer all her emotional needs, and less able to talk to people who can give her another viewpoint on her predicament. The result is that he is able to control her even more.

Most of us have experienced some sort of pangs of jealousy at one time or another, and even in the healthiest of relationships there are sometimes moments when a man or woman feels put out and hurt because their partner has spent all night at a party flirting with someone else. Usually in the cold light of day, after a few cross words, all is forgiven and forgotten.

When a woman lives with an abusive man, however, the situation is different. It is a myth, perpetuated by the abuser, that his jealousy is a sign of his love for his girlfriend or wife. Though at first his jealous outbursts may seem like isolated incidents, they become more and more frequent and unfounded. In an abusive man, jealousy is about control.

An abusive man, albeit subconsciously, uses jealousy to keep his partner 'in her place'. Because his outbursts are unpredictable, she 'walks on eggshells' in fear of him; she is careful not to mention old boyfriends or that her male colleague took her out to lunch. Even close girlfriends pose a threat. So she becomes wary and secretive.

An abuser also makes his partner feel guilty. He will frequently accuse her of dressing too provocatively, or smiling too invitingly:

the implication is that she is a slut, who is just dying to have an affair with any man she meets. Hazel says, 'If we went out anywhere, when we came home the first thing Jimmy would say was: "You made a bloomin' fool of me. I saw you making eyes at such and such a bloke," and I wouldn't know what on earth he was talking about.

'When we went out together, my eyes couldn't leave his face. If my eyes looked one way, he'd accuse me of looking at a man. There was an Australian barman at our local pub, and I used to like talking to him because he had this lovely drawl – I didn't fancy him, but Jimmy really pulled me up on it. He said, "Imagining yourself having it off with him, are you?" You know, he was just stupid, really daft. I mean I wouldn't have dreamed of having an affair anyway. It didn't enter my head.'

Charm Syndrome Man is completely irrational in his jealousy: everyone from the postman to his partner's boss at work comes under suspicion if they threaten to dilute his control over her. One man even stopped his wife from bouncing her four-year-old on her knee – because he was jealous of her spending her affection on him.

An abuser will try to turn his partner against her friends and colleagues by putting them down, or pitting them against each other. Melinda remembers that Trevor was so jealous of her work and her colleagues, even though she had earned enough to put him through university, that he tried to turn her against them by implying that her boss was giving one of her colleagues (a good friend) all the best jobs; although she did not really believe it, it was enough to sow seeds of doubt and make her feel uneasy. 'I had to work,' she says, 'but it was a sort of Catch 22, because the more successful I became, the more insecure he became, and the harder he made it for me.'

On one occasion, he revealed his jealousy in a quite different way, after she had been to the Christmas party given by the firm where she worked. His resentment was compounded by the fact that there were only five women invited to the function, and 1,500 men. 'It was an honour to be asked,' says Melinda. 'I bought a new dress, and a week before I told him, "I have to go to this thing and I will be home by quarter to 12." He was in Guildford that night, he'd been away doing research for his course, and the babysitter said the phone kept on ringing from quarter to 12. Every five minutes he would ring and say, "Is she back?"

'I got back about quarter-past 12 and the girl said the last phone call had been about five minutes before I walked in. The babysitter left, and I went to bed, because I was very tired. The next thing I knew I was being punched. When Trevor found I wasn't home, he had got into the car, and driven down from Guildford to London at ten past midnight, and he went completely berserk. He punched my face – he'd always been very careful not to hit me where it showed before – he hit my head, and I was unrecognisable the next day. And then the children woke up (we had two by now) and it was my daughter who stopped him – by that time he had pushed me down the stairs and I was unconscious on the floor. She just screamed at him to stop and he just stopped. And I came round and said to her, "Go and get your brother, get him out of the house and go next door." And then I got out too. I had said that if he hit me one more time I was going. And so that was it. I never lived with him again.'

Rebecca enrolled at an evening class one night a week – ironically she did so because once they were married this 'amazing man' who 'knew about everything' frequently humiliated her by calling her ignorant. 'One night,' she told me, 'he came to meet me and was in a terrible state. He pushed me into the car and shouted at me all the way home. When we got in, he accused me of having an affair with the teacher and insisted that I was never to go to college again. He kept on at me until four o'clock in the morning and then finally went to sleep, leaving me thinking I really had done something wrong.

'I found out later that he was having an affair with a girl at work – it took me years to get over that. I wanted to leave him then and there, when I found out, but he begged me to forgive him, and he behaved so kindly and reasonably for a while. And there were the children to think of.'

Rebecca's husband, like many abusive men, operated a double standard. He was jealous of her every move, yet it was perfectly okay for *him* to have affairs because that fitted his male image. If an abuser is actually being unfaithful himself, he will often try to transfer the guilt by accusing his wife of doing the same thing. However ridiculous the accusation may be, it serves as a smokescreen for his own infidelities. And, after all, why should he feel guilty if she is behaving in the same way? Furthermore, since an abuser thinks of his wife as a possession, he may even be subconsciously lining up a new woman to control, should his present relationship fail.

Charm Syndrome Man is very often a womaniser. Sally suspected that Guy was having affairs, but he told her she was paranoid for thinking any such thing. Yet she later found out that he belonged to a dating club. Laura suffered even more directly as a result of James's affairs. Like many women whose partners are being unfaithful, she recalls finding out she had a mysterious vaginal infection. 'This is a great joke,' she says. 'I mean, I laugh about this like crazy now, because I remember going to the doctor, and she was saying, "Look. Do you understand that this is sexually transmitted?" and I was saying, "Yes." And she was saying, "Er, what I'm trying to say to you is, either you or your partner has acquired this from somebody else, and both of you have got to take treatment."

'I came home knowing I hadn't been with someone else,' says Laura, yet when she confronted James, suggesting he was having an affair, 'He said, "Nonsense, nonsense, absolute rubbish." And I believed it! But I think you get so worn down that you are prepared to believe just about everything. And yet somewhere you know it's not quite right. He'd had affairs pretty well constantly, though I hadn't known about them at the time.'

Charm Syndrome Man is dependent on his partner, but this often goes unnoticed because he appears so self-assured and because he is so good at controlling his relationships. In reality, his frail self-image requires an adoring woman, and often one such woman is not enough: he may have a steady partner and a stream of disposable mistresses.

Past husbands or boyfriends are just as much a threat to Charm Syndrome Man as imaginary rivals – as Beverley discovered all too soon. 'Dave used to ask me how many lovers I'd had and say, "Oh, I bet you've had loads," and talk about 30 or 40 – unbelievable numbers,' she says. 'He would ask me for figures and I'd say five, or whatever. I said I wasn't really involved with any of them, but this was just as bad as if I had said that I was madly in love with them all. I mean you couldn't win.

'During certain periods, he would wake me up in the morning and say, "Well, what about So-and-So? Did you enjoy it with him? You did, didn't you?" and I would say, "No, I didn't," and he would say, "Are you sure?" And that would happen every morning, with outbursts during the day – not necessarily hitting me, though sometimes he'd slap me across the face and bruise my ribs.'

Dave controlled and confused Beverley by punctuating the abuse with tenderness, begging to be forgiven, telling her he only acted the way he did because he loved her. 'Once it had settled down, those spaces between big instances like black eyes were good – I counted three weeks once when he didn't do anything. That was the record,' she says. 'And that's partly why I stayed. I mean he only cared about these men, ha-ha, because he "loved me so much". He always counteracted with that.'

Sally recalls, 'One day when we were out with my brother and sister-in-law, Guy was filling his car up with petrol and suddenly discovered he didn't have his wallet with him. So I got my bag and wrote out a cheque. The man at the petrol station asked for my address on the back of the cheque (it was in the days before cheque cards) and I automatically put the telephone number too. Then Guy refused to drive out of the station until I explained my actions. He was convinced I fancied the attendant – who was at least 40 years older than me – because I had written down my phone number.

'He insisted on an explanation in front of my brother and his wife and demanded I get the cheque back and write out a new one. After several tense minutes he drove off in a huff and refused to speak to any of us for the rest of the day, even throughout supper.'

Abusive men never forget incidents such as these. They will bring them up again and again over the years, whenever they need to reinforce their current bout of jealousy.

Guy was even jealous of Sally's parents, who wrote to tell her they were coming over to England from their home in New Zealand on a business trip. 'My mum was desperate to see me after three years,' she says. 'After London, they were going on to see some cousins in Jersey for a week, and they wanted me to join them. Guy was outraged at the suggestion that I should abandon him for a whole week. He kept this up for months before the actual event. Believe it or not, he managed to make me feel guilty and his attitude spoiled my reunion with my parents.

'Because I was doing something which he felt excluded him, he got angry over the most stupid things. On the way to the airport to meet my parents, we stopped at our favourite pub for a snack, and – I know it sounds silly – I ordered a salmon and cucumber sandwich. He was so angry and sarcastic about the price. He kept saying, "You always have to have the most extravagant thing! Why can't you have cheese like everybody else?"

'It was all so ridiculous, but at the time I felt so depressed. I was really looking forward to seeing my parents, and he kept putting a dampener on it all. He went on and on about that sandwich all the way to the airport, and even after they had gone home to New Zealand he brought it up again...I realised later it wasn't about the money, it was his way of punishing me, of showing me how angry he was that I had put someone else in front of him.

'Even when I went to Jersey, he phoned every few hours; and if I was out, he wanted to know exactly where I had been and who I had been talking to. He made it all seem very romantic – he couldn't bear me to be away, he cared about me so much that he had to make sure I was okay – but I can see now that he was just checking up on me. Not only was he jealous of my family, but I'm sure he was convinced that I was going to run off with someone else the moment I was away from him.'

Many women tell me their husbands and boyfriends are jealous of their relationships with members of their family. 'He said he wanted me to himself, he didn't want anybody else to have me' is the kind of comment I hear so often. Abusive men are also frequently jealous of their own children, because they divert their partners' attention. This may be one reason why so many men attack their wives during pregnancy. And over and over again I hear stories from women whose husbands refused to attend the birth of their children. Frequently they also overreact when their wives are breastfeeding children. Abusive men often make their partners feel guilty because they have chosen to breastfeed. Some women actually give up breastfeeding because their partners feel ignored in favour of the new arrival; it is simply easier to give in.

Laura's husband James first sexually abused her during the period in which she was breastfeeding her daughter, as if to remind her that *he* should be the centre of her attention. Laura remembers, 'The abuse got worse as the children came along. He felt more and more out of it, or whatever. It certainly got worse then. He always had to centre on *me*. The kids always got shoved to one side. When they were a bit older, he'd tell them to get out of the room, he was talking to *me*. That really used to hurt me.' She recalled a time when James refused to let her go and watch the children in their nursery-school nativity play. He had refused to go, because he wanted to watch a TV documentary, and he insisted she should stay with *him* rather than be with the children.

Another woman I met told how her husband was so jealous he even accused her of having sex with her nine-year-old son, a suspicion which totally disgusted her.

Some abusers are even jealous of objects if they seem to threaten their monopoly over their partners' affections. Hazel's husband

Jimmy noted anything she particularly loved. 'In the next dispute,' she says, 'it would be destroyed. For instance I love sewing and one day I said to someone in his presence, "I love my sewing machine." Some time afterwards when he was in a childlike temper, he picked it up above his head and slammed it to the floor, and of course it broke. It was as if he was jealous of an inanimate object.'

This is all too typical. Many abusers will destroy family photographs and personal possessions with sentimental value in order to undermine and punish a woman. One woman I counselled told me that her partner ripped up photographs of their new baby in front of her simply because he felt there were more pictures of her family than of his. Another woman was overjoyed when she received a major promotion at work...until her husband tore up letters of congratulations from her friends and family. For her, that one act was a culmination of years of put-downs, verbal abuse and jealousy. Tearing up her letters was the last straw and she left.

## 'He tracked my every move'

Since I wrote the first edition of this book, advances in technology have afforded abusers an arsenal of high-tech gadgets with which to control and terrorise women. Where in the past an abuser may have phoned 'his woman' every half an hour to ensure she didn't leave the house, now, he might use cameras, spyware or GPS software to put her under surveillance. Placing a tracker on a woman's car is relatively easy to do and allows abusers to know whether she deviates from the routine he expects of her. Even when a woman's abuser is at work or away from home, there is no escaping his control – it becomes impossible for her to lead an independent life. One woman told me: 'Somehow he would know if I hadn't come straight back home after dropping the children at school. He would demand to know where I had been and verbally abuse me until I told him. In the end, I stopped doing anything – it felt like he had spies everywhere, but of course it was the car.'

Another woman told me her husband fixed a tracker onto her car so he would know where she had parked it, and then go and move it. 'You've lost it!' he would say. 'You must have just forgotten where you parked.' Imagine the psychological impact of being forced to doubt yourself like this, again and again.

Of course, technology – and the communication and connections it brings – can be a powerful tool to reduce a woman's isolation and may enable her to access support for the first time. The 'Get Help' pages of Refuge's website are accessed by almost half a million individuals per year. Yet technology use may also lead to unintended consequences – for example, tracking women through apps on smart phones is common.

In what seems like a romantic gesture, a perpetrator might buy his partner a brand new iPhone or laptop – it may be months before she realises he has fitted it with technology that sends her Google searches or her text messages to him. One woman told me: 'He knew things that he definitely could not have known unless he was spying on me – stuff I had sent on my computer, which he didn't have access to. It slowly dawned on me that he must have some other way – some kind of technology.' Spyware software like this can easily be bought online – some is even marketed as a way of keeping an eye on your 'cheating wife' or troublesome teenager. When it comes to technology, the possibilities for abuse are endless.

## 'He always put me down'

Guy never missed an opportunity to undermine Sally's self-confidence and make her feel inadequate. He nagged her, constantly picking up on anything he could interpret as a fault in her character, gradually eroding her sense of self. 'It was almost as if he was on the lookout for flaws in my character,' says Sally. 'He would pick up on the most trivial things.

'For example, one day I gave my mother a quick ring to see how she was getting on. Guy was peeling potatoes for supper and listening to *The Archers,* so I went into the hall to phone. When I finished the conversation, I went back into the kitchen, to be greeted by Guy saying disapprovingly, "Do you realise you just said 'okay' *14* times?" I sensed that his motives for saying this were negative, but I couldn't work out why he did it. I felt really embarrassed, humiliated and so ashamed, and then before I knew it I was promising to watch my "okays" in future.'

Taken as an isolated incident, it seems very trivial, yet by this stage of their relationship Sally was exhausted by Guy's constant need to put her down. His unceasing criticism of the way she looked and behaved and thought wore her down like water dripping on a stone. Not only did he criticise her, but he was continually disparaging about her friends and colleagues at work, even her intelligence. This endless undermining of her personality kept him firmly in control. Sally began to be more and more submissive, doubting her own opinions and relying on his.

Many women suffer such acute humiliation, degradation and bewilderment at the hands of their abusers that their self-esteem takes a severe battering. Instead of seeing themselves as worthwhile, important and valid people, they feel inferior, because their personality has been consistently mocked and attacked. They feel unattractive, usually because their partners have told them they are. They feel worthless, unwanted, insecure; they doubt their ability to make relationships work; they are unsure of their judgement and continually apologise for their actions. They say, 'If only I hadn't done this,' or 'I wish I were different.'

Many of the abused women I talk to are highly intelligent, respected, professional people, who are perfectly capable of trusting their own judgement and making decisions at high levels, yet in their personal relationships these same women often feel nervous and unsure of themselves as a direct effect of their partner's controlling behaviour. It is hard enough for women to have high self-esteem anyway in a male-dominated world. Some women already feel vulnerable – and when women are abused as well, they feel doubly worthless and insecure. To have and maintain self-esteem you need to feel in control of your life.

Trevor would constantly tell Melinda that she was 'hopeless'. 'He'd say, "When you met me, you thought you were somebody special, didn't you? I bet you don't now, do you?" and I used to say, "No." I think I underestimated the power of the verbal and emotional abuse at the time, the things he used to say to me. He'd call me slag, whore, bitch, dog – you name it, very denigrating names,' she says.

Hazel, too, says, 'Jimmy used to call me slag, trollop, horrible things, because he knew it upset me, that it was the one thing I couldn't get hardened to.' Hazel had been brought up in a warm, happy family and made friends easily, yet by the time she left Jimmy, she felt so physically bruised, psychologically scarred and sexually humiliated that, she told me: 'I felt no one would want me after what he had put me through. He destroyed all my self-confidence. He told me nobody liked me, that people only put up with me because I was with him – you know, that I lived in his shadow. I felt drained, just drained. As if I was nothing, as if I was worthless.'

'You're no good for anyone' is the kind of put-down women report to me time and time again. Laura told me that, in one sickening telephone call after they had split up, James had snarled at her, 'I dragged you up out of the gutter. Why don't you do everyone a favour and go and kill yourself?' Then he hung up.

One woman I spoke to told me that her husband frequently acted as if she didn't even exist. In one such instance, she had spent all day painting and decorating their home, not even stopping to have anything to eat. When her husband came back from work that evening, having stopped to have a drink with colleagues on the way, he brought in a takeaway kebab for himself – and nothing for her, despite the fact that he knew she would not have had dinner without him. Like most women who recount such stories, she was embarrassed at the triviality of it, yet this was only one example amid numerous others which had left her feeling hurt that she had sunk so far in her husband's estimation that he barely even acknowledged her existence.

This woman's husband also attacked her self-confidence by being cruel about her appearance. She had a scar on her neck from a growth which had been removed when she was ten. 'People say they don't notice it, but I know it's there,' she says, 'and my husband knew I had a really bad inferiority complex about it. When I first met him he would say, "Oh, I don't notice", but later he would say things like "When I first saw your scar it made me want to be sick."'

Hazel knew what it was like to have her appearance constantly criticised. 'Apart from telling me that I was useless at everything, that I was no good,' she says, 'Jimmy used to say that I was fat and horrible, that I was lucky to have him as nobody else would look at me. After a while I really started to believe it. I stopped caring about what I looked like, basically because what was the point? I never went anywhere and I never saw anyone. The only person I saw was him, and if I did make the effort and try to look nice, put a bit of make-up on or something, he'd say, "What the hell are you all dressed up for? Who have you had round here?"'

Dave used terror tactics to humiliate and frighten Beverley in order to undermine her personality. One day, she told me: 'He came home and he came up to me and said, "Do you love me?" and I said "Yes," and I went to put my arms around him, and he thumped me in the stomach and just kept hitting and kicking me, kicking and hitting. He hadn't done that before. I was just thinking, "My God, this is it, he really is going to kill me now – what can I do?"

'We were in a top-floor flat so I couldn't get outside, and he dragged me right across the flat by my hair into the kitchen, then he got out the kitchen knife, and I thought, "Oh, *no!*" Even though I thought he might not mean to kill me, it is very easy to kill somebody with a blade like that and he was angry.

'I kept yelling, "*I love you! I love you!*" as if that was the answer and that would stop him. And I put out my hands and got my fingers cut – but do you know what he was doing? He was cutting my hair off! My hair came down to my waist, and he cut it all off. And then he just sat there saying, "You're ugly now." Because, you see, he didn't want me to be attractive, and he hacked my hair off so that it was one inch long. You don't realise how easily hair comes off with a sharp knife – just two cuts and that was it.

'Every time I saw myself in the mirror I looked so ugly, I felt this great sense of despair. I felt worthless, that I must be a really bad person to make him do this to me.'

By deliberately damaging Beverley's self-esteem, Dave could make himself feel superior to her, and therefore more entitled to be in control. Ironically, though, the haircutting incident drove Beverley away. 'Despite the sense of humiliation, I had enough strength to leave,' she says. 'I knew the situation was beyond my control.'

An abuser will often use social abuse to undermine his partner, humiliating her in front of friends and family, often in subtle ways. As one woman explained, 'When my husband's sister and her boyfriend came to visit, he brought them in a cup of tea and cakes and biscuits, but he left me out. He didn't give me a cup and he never offered me a cake.'

Laura told me that James would make her feel she had behaved foolishly in front of his friends. 'I would be blamed for having said the wrong thing, which to me wouldn't have seemed like the wrong thing in any way. He would say I had put my foot in it over something which I didn't think was justified at all. He made me feel small and insignificant. He liked to put me down in front of other people, sort of saying, "What on earth is that you're wearing?" and "You don't know what you are talking about" and "You don't understand." Anything to make me feel small.'

The point about this sort of social abuse is that an abuser is always in control, unlike his partner, who never knows how he will behave towards her in front of other people.

Trevor would always pick an argument or try to degrade Melinda, just before she went off to an important meeting. 'He would find some excuse to put me down, to upset me, to be aggressive and abusive so

I would always arrive feeling very unsure of myself, very insecure and very, very weak,' she remembers. 'I would be needing to communicate with people in a position of responsibility, with a lot to express, and all I would feel like doing was sitting down and crying. It was such a horrible feeling, it actually prevented me from communicating with other people, and communicating about my work.'

Jimmy, like many abusive men, undermined Hazel in another, very powerful way: he attacked her role as a mother. 'He'd say, "You're bringing up our son all wrong,"' she says. '"He's soft, he's pathetic." I suppose deep down I knew it was a game that he was playing with me, and nothing to do with my son, or anything I did with him. But he made me feel as if I was a failure at my marriage and I wasn't a good mother – as if I wasn't a good woman, I suppose.'

James tried to control Laura by undermining her role as mother, even after they had separated. He went so far as actually to ring up her children's school, saying, 'Laura's mad, she's drunk, she's taking drugs, she's not a reasonable mother. She's an alcoholic and a whore.' Another time, he promised to pay the school fees; not only did he fail to pay them, but, says Laura, 'He told the bursar he'd given me the money and I'd spent it. It was a new school and they didn't know me. The bursar rang me up and said, "I'm sorry your daughters can't come back to school. I've been told you've got the money and you haven't paid the bill." And I said, "It's not true, I haven't got it." He said, "Well, look, I'm awfully sorry, but I can't enter into that sort of thing," and of course he couldn't. I mean it's no good saying, "It's not true," is it?'

## 'I thought I must be going crazy'

Melinda felt so manipulated, confused and disorientated by her husband's abusive behaviour that she compared him to the husband in the film *Gaslight*. 'I felt he was trying to convince me that I was insane,' she says.

The film *Gaslight* starred Ingrid Bergman, with Charles Boyer as the husband who seemed so romantic and charming, while all the time he was manipulating his wife into thinking she was going crazy. His technique was to hide jewellery, then accuse her of losing it, or take pictures from the wall and insist she had removed them. He would swing from anger to charm, confusing and frightening her so much that she began to believe she really was to blame. Because he convinced her that he still loved her and would look after her, she became more and more dependent on him, unable to see that *he* was the cause of her misery.

Well, that is pure fiction, and the Charles Boyer character was a calculating villain, yet in an unconscious way Charm Syndrome Man often behaves in a very similar fashion, controlling through manipulation.

Trevor actually did behave like the Charles Boyer character on occasions: he would deliberately hide things in order to confuse Melinda. On one occasion her son caught him doing it and told his mother. 'He had seen his father move the sugar basin from one place to another,' says Melinda. 'All the while he was laughing and smiling to himself, then he came into the living room, demanding, "Who moved this, then?" and started a big row.'

Another of Charm Syndrome Man's techniques is to imply that his partner is imagining things. One of the few places Rebecca felt she could relax and escape from Ralph's nagging over every little detail was the garden. When he was at work, she would spend hours outside, nurturing plants from cuttings. 'It was a real labour of love,' she says. 'Although Ralph didn't share my love of flowers he did help by mowing the grass regularly. But it used to sadden me that every single time he did this he would "accidentally" chop off the flower heads – usually the best ones – by just not being careful enough when he went along by the beds. To start with I used to think it was genuinely by mistake. Gradually it dawned on me that this was no mistake. Not only was it getting to be a habit, but he would laugh in my face as well if I mentioned it, and say I was mad.'

The abuse of Helen Titchener at the hands of her husband, Rob, on the BBC Radio soap *The Archers* shone a light on this particularly insidious technique of control. To ensure he could always keep an eye on Helen, Rob muscled in on her job at the family farm shop. Soon, the stock orders were muddled – thanks to 'silly' Helen. According to Rob, Helen – who was pregnant at the time – had even absentmindedly scalded her little boy in the bath. The more Rob built up this narrative of forgetfulness, fragility and hormonal hysteria, the more convinced Helen became that it was true – particularly when he picked on her past eating disorder as proof of her feeble-mindedness. He even persuaded her to visit a psychiatrist.

Like Rob Titchener, Guy could be caring, loving and tender towards Sally at times, yet emotionally abusive at others. As a result of this see-sawing behaviour, she says, 'I became very, very confused. At times I thought the abuse hadn't really happened, that I'd imagined it. There was a period of time when I didn't know who I was, I didn't know what was right, what was wrong, what was happening. I wanted to leave, but he convinced me that I was responsible for the problems, so I'd try even harder to make the relationship work.'

The Charles Boyer character in *Gaslight* was a charmer, cleverly alternating romance with anger, so that his wife never knew what to expect. It is the kind of mental torment used so successfully by torturers and terrorists who know that they can keep their prisoners compliant by frightening and disorienting them with rapidly changing moods and situations. A well-known Gestapo technique involved wearing down and confusing prisoners with torture followed by kindness. Charm Syndrome Man, on an unconscious level, does the same thing. The more the woman doubts herself and her sanity, and the more uncertain she becomes, the easier it is for her abuser to keep her under control.

Melinda described her state of mind towards the end of her marriage: 'I think the confusion was the worst thing,' she says. 'It makes one kind of paralysed. And you keep on thinking if you try hard enough, maybe it will change.' Her account of her confusion is very typical of the way many women feel living with Charm Syndrome Man. 'I think the main effect was that I no longer knew what was real and what was not real,' she says. 'I began to lose my ability and confidence to make those kinds of assessments. I always felt that I had been a relatively strong and independent person before I met Trevor, and so I found it difficult to accept that I was in this situation, that these strange things which didn't make sense were happening to me.'

Her predicament was heightened by the response of friends and colleagues. 'They had always known me as a fairly strong-minded person who always spoke her mind, who was very indignant about violence and abuse, and I had always seen myself that way too. So they couldn't understand.

'Sometimes I would see my friends and I would be in pieces and I would want to talk about it and be comforted and get it all out, but I found it very difficult to describe what was happening because it was so incredibly violent and aggressive and frightening, and yet I was still with the man. So the attitude of my friends was: "If it's really that bad, why are you still there?" Because I didn't know the answer to that either it confused me even more, so in the end I suppose I would make light of it, because I couldn't answer the question.

'I find it much easier to understand now, but at the time I was completely confused, so I lost my base within myself. There was a period when I didn't know who I was, and I didn't know what was happening. I was so confused, and I was frightened that I had nothing of myself to fall back on, nothing that was solid and true, so I wasn't in a position to leave.

'Trevor could just switch from being lovely one moment into this kind of unpredictable, very aggressive person the next, and that was something I found confusing and frightening: not knowing when it was going to happen. When we went to bed together, I never knew whether I was going to be loved or whether I was going to be ignored, to be hit or shouted at, or frightened or put down or criticised or kicked. I just didn't know what was going to happen.

'I became very tense and anxious because he had such power, really the power that could affect me, because when somebody you love is very nice one moment and explosive and critical the next, you never know what to expect, so you can't ever quite relax. You are always frightened of a backlash. I had always been used to having a certain amount of power over what happened to me, and here I was in a situation totally without power. I had times of being incredibly angry, and wanting revenge. I was shocked by the hatred I felt towards him. Yet, two weeks after that, he could make me feel full of love and care and tenderness towards him, and that confused me a lot.

'We would have very calm times and then there were the most enormous upheavals, and it was terrifying. It was incredibly extreme, and then somehow it would go, it would dissipate. I'd be really shocked that it had happened, whereas Trevor's attitude was that either it hadn't happened, that I was imagining it, or that it was normal, and that I was the one who was unbalanced in thinking his behaviour was wrong or extreme.'

In her confusion, it was all too easy for Trevor to manipulate her into believing that she was overreacting or simply being neurotic.

Hazel likened her sense of confusion to being 'under a spell'. 'It's like they've got possession over you. You believe everything they tell you. Jimmy would say, "I only beat you because I love you. If I didn't love you, I wouldn't hit you", and at the time I believed him. I used to doubt my own sanity a lot. Jimmy would say that I was frigid, that I was ugly, all kinds of things, to put me down. He knew that I never felt attractive, and he would knock me down. But then the next time he would say that I was beautiful and that I was the best mother in the world, and I was the best wife in the world. Then, in the next breath, I was the worst.'

'One of the biggest problems was the confusion of it all,' agrees Laura. 'There would be a pattern of enormous calm and togetherness and empathy and love, then there would be periods of conflict. James could be very sarcastic, very snide, very cold and very threatening. He would use his words like powerful weapons. Then he would be gentle and considerate. It was rather like walking on a volcano. Sometimes it's safe, sometimes it isn't. That confusion gave him all the control.'

One of the major weapons in Charm Syndrome Man's arsenal is this ability to be a Dr Jekyll and Mr Hyde. He confuses his partner by being abusive one minute, charming the next, blinding her to the bad times, making her forgive him, feel sorry for him, give him another chance. The most predictable thing about Charm Syndrome Man is his unpredictability. I have even heard of men turning up at refuges with flowers and chocolates. They send love letters, expensive presents – anything to win back the woman and convince her that everything will change.

Hazel says, 'Jimmy would just keep saying he was sorry, that he couldn't bear the idea of living without me. Sometimes I'd leave, and go and stay with my mother, but he'd come round and say he'd seen the light, he realised what he'd done. And I'd think, "Oh, he *has* seen it." I used to think he was really sorry, but the minute I got back he was blaming me again. I just felt that he'd conned me again, which made me feel stupid. I felt like an idiot for falling for it, but you've no idea how convincing he can be.

'And I really did want him to be like he used to be, like the Jimmy I first met. And there were lovely times. Saturdays were always special to us. I'd put on a dress and make a special dinner, and he'd do the table. We'd spoil each other. For a long time the good times outweighed the outbursts.'

Not only are they confused themselves, but most women I talk to tell me that their desperation is compounded by the fact that to friends and neighbours their abusers appear to be such good-natured chaps. To the outside world they are still charmers. Who is going to believe that behind closed doors they are making life hell for their partners? The reaction is likely to be: the woman must be crazy!

Manipulating a woman to doubt her own experiences is a particularly cruel technique – and one in which society colludes. Women are routinely disbelieved when they report sexual or domestic violence. We know that 85 per cent of domestic violence victims sought help from professionals five times before they got effective support.[8] Her Majesty's Inspectorate of Constabulary has found that 26 per cent of sexual offences reported to the police are not even recorded as crimes.[9] Imagine you have been raped by your abusive husband. When you protest the next day, he tells you there's been a mistake – 'You said "yes", like you always do,' he says. You know you didn't, but he insists and he has turned on the charm – you see a glimpse of the man you fell in love with, and you want to avoid another barrage of abuse. It is easier to believe him, especially because you fear the police wouldn't take you seriously anyway. Perpetrators render women unreliable witnesses to their own lives – and every time a woman's testimony is dismissed as untrue, or exaggerated, or 'not such a big deal', it bolsters their abuse.

Not only does Charm Syndrome Man convince others that he is the good guy, but he cannot bear to admit to himself that he has any faults. He may not be aware of it, but it is very important to him to be seen as the perfect husband and provider. 'The most irritating, frustrating thing,' says Melinda, 'was that other people always saw Trevor as Mr Nice Guy. Whenever we were in company, he was tender, he was interested, he was a really nice bloke, and very, very few people had any indication of what was going on. My own family to this day doesn't believe any of this, and they think that he is a really nice bloke. I mean, when I told my sister I had to call the police out, she said, "Are you sure you didn't do something?" My family would say, "Trevor loves you and he wants to take care of you, you know. Are you sure you are not making a big issue about it?" And you wonder if that's what you are doing.'

When Laura and James were splitting up, she remembers the situation with anger: 'He used to take my particular friends out to lunch and pour his heart out and say how miserable he was. He made a wonderful victim – he's very appealing. They were quite often people he'd been very rude to before, but he managed to win them over. I thought that if I heard one more person say "Poor James", I would scream.

'They would say things like "James is really unhappy. Perhaps you should try giving him more attention", or "He really does love you, you know. Why are you so hard on him?" This was the man who was bullying me and hitting me to the point that I was a jittering wreck. When I heard the key in the door I'd start thinking, "God, he's coming back. What kind of mood is he going to be in?" And my friends were telling me I should try harder!

'He would always appear to be a passionate believer in freedom from oppression. My mouth would hang open and my eyes would widen when I heard him talking to our friends about human rights. It was sheer hypocrisy. If people had known what he was doing to me on an individual level... He was such a good actor. If he walked in here now, you'd probably be charmed by him. He liked to play Mr Nice Guy, Mr Wonderful, Mr Liberal...'

Charm Syndrome Man often distorts reality even further (albeit unconsciously) by telling his partner's friends and family that she is hysterical or paranoid. He may even threaten to have her admitted to a psychiatric hospital, using blackmail to get what he wants. When Laura threatened divorce, she says, 'James knew he wouldn't get custody of the children so he would say, "I will have you declared insane, you're not fit. You're just sitting around crying all the time." Well, at that stage I *was* sitting around crying.'

Just as charm is the abuser's greatest weapon when it comes to winning over family and friends, and confusing his partner, it is also his trump card should the police become alerted to his violence. On one occasion when Jimmy became so violent that Hazel ran from the house and came to Refuge, he actually went to the police and told them that she was depressed to the point of suicide, and that she had run away with the baby. He convinced them that he was afraid for her safety and that of the child.

The police went to see Hazel's sister – one of the few people who knew the truth – and she told them about his violent and unpredictable behaviour. If she had run away, she said, it would be because she was in fear for her life. The policeman's attitude was 'But he seems like a very reasonable young man.'

## 'I felt so alone'

As time went on, Melinda began to feel very alone in her relationship with Trevor. Almost without realising it, she had cut herself off from her friends, relying more and more on him for everything.

This was no accident. Charm Syndrome Man controls his partner by isolating her from family and friends and outside interests. *He* must be the focus of her attention. Anyone who attempts to share her love and affection is a threat. In a healthy, happy relationship, there is give and take, and both partners feel free to see friends and family, to work and pursue their own interests. But when a woman lives with an abusive man, he is the one in control, he makes all the plans and all the rules. He will encourage his partner to devote all of her time and energy to him, using his charm to make his demands seem romantic: who needs anyone else, when you have each other?

'Looking back,' says Sally, talking about the early days with Guy, 'I can see it was a sort of suffocation, but he made me feel there was no need for anyone else, we were so wrapped up in each other – that seemed to be enough. He told me I was special and beautiful and all those things, and that he didn't want to share me with anyone else.'

Charm Syndrome Man will do everything in his power to discourage friends and activities which take his partner away from the home. He may refuse to allow her to take a driving test if she cannot drive, or refuse access to the car if she can. If she wants to take a job, he will use every argument he can muster to prevent her, even if he has to accuse her of being a bad mother, deserting her children to go out to work, or put her down and ridicule her for thinking she is capable of taking a job at all.

One woman I met told me how her husband used more subtle tactics. 'I was going for an interview for a job at five o'clock,' she says. 'We were out shopping and time was getting on so I asked him to pick the kids up from school, and meet me back at Sainsbury's so we could get home and I'd have time to get ready for the interview.

'He went off, and I must have sat outside Sainsbury's waiting for over an hour – I'd got about eight bags – and eventually I had to walk about half a mile to catch a bus. I couldn't get a cab, I wasn't allowed to spend that sort of money. By the time I got home, after waiting for a bus, it was hours later, and I'd missed the interview.

'He was asleep in front of the TV and the kids hadn't even been fed when I got in. He said he'd had a look in the shop and couldn't see me, so he'd just come home. But I knew why he'd done it. I said, "It's because I was going for an interview for a job, isn't it? You're trying to drag me down." As I sat down he started slapping me and throwing things and screaming.'

What once seemed to be a demonstration of love can turn into a kind of possessiveness. 'Don't go, stay here with me – I miss you when you're away' is pretty irresistible at first, and, after all, it seems such a small thing to cancel an evening class, or a night out with a friend, but invariably these 'one-off' occasions occur again and again, until the woman begins to feel very alone. But precisely because each occasion does seem to be a 'one-off', she is often unaware of what is happening, until her isolation is extreme.

Early on in Sally's relationship with Guy she moved out of the house she was sharing with two girlfriends, and into a flat with him. One day one of her former flatmates rang to say she had an extra ticket for the ballet and asked her to come. Sally knew Guy was giving an extra tutorial that evening, so she accepted. 'When Guy rang later in the day,' says Sally, 'I told him, and there was a stony silence at the other end of the line. Then he said, "Do you mean to say you are going?" When I said that I was, he said "I see" in a voice that sounded both hurt and accusing at the same time. He put the phone down on me and I spent the rest of the day feeling nervy and uncomfortable.

'When I was getting ready at the flat, he came back and said he'd cancelled the tutorial. He was very cold towards me and answered me in monosyllables. I finally felt I had to ring my friend and say I couldn't come. It was right at the last minute and I felt so embarrassed with my lame excuses. When I had finished the call, Guy said, "I'm glad you got your priorities right." It sounded like a warning – a sort of threat. I was bitterly angry, but I kept quiet, to keep the peace. Shortly afterwards he was all love and attentiveness; it was all right again. He made me feel it had been such a little sacrifice to make for our relationship. I dismissed it at the time – though, looking back, part of me felt that something was wrong.' Much later, Sally found out that while she was cutting herself off from the outside world and devoting all her energies to Guy, he was off having affairs with other women.

Another woman I talked to faced hostility whenever she wanted to go out with friends. On one occasion she asked her husband if she could go round to a friend's for a 'girls' night in'. Since he normally grumbled if she wanted to do anything without him, she was surprised when he said yes, of course she could go. When the evening arrived, she cooked the supper and got the children ready for bed, before getting dressed. 'I was so excited because I hadn't been out for months,' she told me. 'And I was so pleased that he hadn't said a word about it since the time I asked him. I'd had my hair done and looked out a nice dress to wear. I went up to change and put on my make-up. He came in and gave me a cuddle and my heart really lifted. I kissed the children goodbye and went out of the front door. The next thing I remember is that I was hit by water. My hair was clinging to my head and my dress was sopping. I looked up and there he was leaning out of the bedroom window with an empty bucket. He was laughing and he said, "Where do you think you're going then?" I went back into the house and cried.

'I was so hurt and angry and humiliated that I think I would have left him at that moment if it hadn't been for the children and the fact that I had no job, and nowhere to go.'

Beverley had a fairly independent lifestyle before she met Dave and had been used to having her own friends, but she admits that when they started going out together she neglected them for Dave, because she was so wrapped up in the relationship, and was flattered that he always wanted her to himself. Here we see how insidiously the normal features of a romantic relationship can blur into the beginning of controlling behaviour. Wanting to be together can lead to the man isolating the woman. This is one reason why abusive behaviour can be so hard to predict when a relationship begins. Beverley, however, after her marriage made a conscious effort to pick up again with her friends.

'Looking back on it,' she says, 'when I started breaking out and having interests, that was when Dave started getting cross.' She recalls the time she joined a badminton club with a friend, having already asked Dave if he would like to join. He had said no. 'When I came in,' she remembers, 'it was only half-past nine or something, not late, but later than he thought I should be, and he really went mad, and this was the first time I was frightened.' Beverley told me she was subjected to a complete interrogation: 'Where have you been? What have you been doing? You can't have been playing badminton all this time. Don't you realise that I worry?'

She told him that she had had to wait for a court, to which he replied, 'I don't know why you go anyway. I don't do this to you – I don't go out.' Beverley continues, 'I said, "I wish you would. Go out with a friend." But his answer was "I don't need to – you're enough for me and obviously I'm not enough for you." He was really very, very angry – he was beating his fists on the table, and I could see the violence within him – he was holding it back.'

Shocked and frightened at this new behaviour, Beverley rang her mother-in-law from the kitchen. This was a woman with whom she had a close relationship, yet her response was: 'Well, my darling, why do you go to these things? Why don't you stay at home with your husband? That's your place.'

Social abuse is an important part of the abuser's armoury. Not only will he try to keep his partner at home, but he will also discourage callers. If friends come to the house, he will create an atmosphere, so that in the end, however angry she may feel, the woman finds it less embarrassing simply to discourage visitors altogether. 'If I had friends to the house,' says Hazel, 'Jimmy would behave in the most disgusting manner possible. I remember once I invited one of the girls I worked with at the hairdresser's round for a drink and something to eat. Jimmy refused to sit in the same room as us for a start. He sat in the front room so we had to sit in the kitchen, and he sat there with the television on really loudly. And when I took his dinner through – a perfectly nice dinner – he brought it back in and said, "You don't expect me to eat this muck, do you?" and threw it on the floor in front of my friend. Can you imagine how embarrassed I was?'

Finally, Hazel says, 'I just stopped inviting people to the house, because I didn't know how he would behave. I began to get panicky when people called. I mean I really did, I began to shake and I just wanted them to go. That cut me off as well. And I didn't go and see anybody because I wasn't allowed out anyway. I felt I had nobody.'

Rebecca told me that, as time went on, the outings to the theatre and to favourite restaurants fell by the wayside, and she and Ralph hardly had any visitors. She explained, 'In theory he said he liked people to come over, but he had this way of making them feel so uncomfortable that I found it embarrassing.' After Ralph retired, her sense of isolation was greater than ever, because he demanded her constant attention, and became less willing than ever to entertain or go to see friends. She even discovered that if people called while she was out, inviting them to dinner or to parties, Ralph would simply decline, without consulting her or even telling her about the invitation. Only when she happened to bump into friends who would say 'Sorry you couldn't make it' did she realise what had been happening.

Families pose a huge threat to Charm Syndrome Man, because if a woman has a close bond with her parents or her brothers and sisters, it jeopardises his complete control over her. He will go to great lengths to discourage her from seeing her family, embarrassing them if they call or trying to poison his partner against them. By putting other people down, he believes he is elevating himself in his partner's eyes.

Though an abuser rarely focuses his violence on anyone outside his immediate family circle, it is not uncommon for him to beat up his partner's mother, her sister or any relative who is close enough to be viewed as an extension of his partner. The result is that the woman feels so frightened for that person that she would rather suffer loneliness and isolation than subject a loved one to danger.

One woman told me that one night her husband started kicking her while her mother was visiting from abroad. When she heard her screams, her mother came rushing into the room. 'My husband got hold of her,' says the woman, 'and said, "*You!* You have no right to interfere – this is my house", and got hold of her arm – she was 67 then – dragged her upstairs by the arm to her bedroom and locked her in it.

'Then he came back down and started hitting me again…the next day he told my mother she had to be out of the house. He made her change her air ticket and leave early, which was awful for my poor old mum. And from then on it was terrible, just one row after another, with him accusing me of putting my family first, loving my family more than him. The rows would go into the night – two, three in the morning.' The result of all this was that out of fear for her mother's safety, and shame at her witnessing her husband's behaviour, the woman began to discourage visits.

When a woman lives with an abusive man, she is the one who must alter her lifestyle, and what he is permitted to do does not necessarily apply to her. Charm Syndrome Man frequently sees his own friends, and goes out on his own, leaving his partner at home, increasing her sense of isolation.

Control through isolation serves another purpose: if a woman has no contact with friends and relations, who is she going to tell when the abuse gets too much? As Melinda says, 'I had nobody.' Furthermore, Trevor had warned her, 'If you tell anybody about what I do to you, I'll kill you', and she had every reason to believe him. The woman is caught in a vicious circle. Her isolation makes her more and more dependent on her partner. She has no one outside the relationship who can give an objective view, she's cut off from sources of support, so that if her partner beats her, humiliates and degrades her, and then tells her she deserves it, she begins to believe him. His are the only views she hears. There is no one else to shed light on the situation. So she begins to believe she is to blame, that she is somehow causing him to be abusive.

To the abusive man, anything that increases his victim's independence is a threat that must be neutralised. Isolation is a key weapon in wearing his partner down. The less interaction she has with the outside world, the more dependent she becomes, and the more she believes what he says about her is true – including that she is to blame for his abuse. Even for women who work, their activities are controlled – they must arrive home by a certain time and only speak to people whom he deems appropriate. As an abused woman's isolation increases, so does her loneliness. Cut off from family, friends and colleagues, she becomes less able to assess objectively her situation, and the perpetrator's grip is tightened.

## 'His anger cut like a knife'

Charm Syndrome Man can control his partner through anger, or by withdrawing affection and attention. He behaves like a dictator, using his anger to get his way, to intimidate his partner. A man does not have to shout, or hit his partner: he can show his anger by being moody or sulky. So much so that his moods dominate the whole atmosphere in the household. Often such mood swings are so subtle that they go undetected by others who are present – but his partner knows, and she feels wounded, humiliated, often frightened. To her, his anger is as devastating as a slap in the face.

Beverley told me that on several occasions after Dave had been sulking for days and refusing to talk to her, they would meet up with mutual friends for a drink, and he would be telling jokes and chatting as though nothing had happened – except that he would avoid any eye contact with her. 'I felt as though he was having a good time with everyone else but me,' she says. 'I felt excluded. But no one else would have noticed. I'd keep trying to get him to look at me, but he wouldn't. I used to feel so tense and edgy. So I would just stand there, not saying anything, while everyone thought Dave was such good fun, and I was really boring.'

Another woman I met never knew what was going to send her partner into a mood that would consume the entire household. 'It sounds so silly now, but I used to get cross with myself for not having warned friends and family against mentioning whatever ridiculous thing he was angry about at the time. I remember, my dad once innocently mentioned something about our Christmas tree, which sent him into a mood that lasted two weeks. Once Dad had gone, he had tears streaming down his face – he said my father thought everything he did wasn't good enough. He wouldn't talk to me or our daughter for days and days. And I thought "What was I thinking? I should have told Dad not to mention the Christmas tree!" I was constantly consumed by how I could pacify him, how I could prevent something totally insignificant setting him off. It was so draining.'

Other men use anger to embarrass their partners in front of other people – so that rather than be made to look foolish, they turn down invitations and unwittingly comply with their partners' wishes by spending all their time with them.

Sally told me of a time when Guy started a row in the middle of a crowded restaurant, then walked out – leaving her scarlet with embarrassment – and with no money to pay the bill. Another time, they had had an argument on the way to a concert, which he tried to continue once the orchestra had started playing. Aware of people's irritation around her she whispered, 'Please can we talk about it later?', but his reaction was to slam his programme loudly onto his seat and storm out while everyone was telling him to shush. She was left squirming, to find her own way home after the concert.

Sometimes social abuse is more subtle. I supported a woman whose husband would allow her to throw dinner parties but then reduce her to tears just before the guests arrived, criticising the way she looked and what she was cooking. As soon as the doorbell rang, she would disappear upstairs to compose herself, and hear him laughing and joking with their guests. Of course, as much as she tried to behave 'normally', she would spend the evening anticipating more anger and abuse. He would be the life and soul of the party, and she would be withdrawn and quiet – leaving friends to form the opinion that she was the grumpy one. Most of us get angry at some time or another, say things we do not mean or act petulantly. But the difference between an 'ordinary' row and an abusive situation is that an abuser uses anger regularly as a controlling device. He doesn't just 'fly off the handle sometimes'; his anger is part of a larger pattern of behaviour. A woman needs to ask herself whether she can live with the rows, whether they are just blow-ups that are soon forgotten or whether they are one factor in a whole set of incidents which make her feel unhappy, frightened or demeaned. For example, is he also jealous and dominant, does he try to isolate her from other people, does he frequently try to make her look foolish and stupid?

She should also ask herself whether her partner's anger is directed *only* at her. An abusive man is usually capable of keeping his temper with his own friends, or colleagues at work, but at home he believes that he is entitled to use anger to keep his partner in check or to get his own way. He is not some inarticulate, inadequate person who is unable to communicate with others. Charm

Syndrome Man has very good coping skills. In fact, he is highly manipulative and is often capable of lying and distorting reality to suit his own needs. Contrary to what a lot of psychologists believe, this is not the behaviour of someone with 'limited coping skills'. The problem is that Charm Syndrome Man is almost *too good* at coping. What he needs to do is unlearn some of these coping skills, that is, unlearn his controlling behaviour. An abuser denies his partner the right to her own opinions. He sees her not as her own person, but as an extension of himself, so if she disagrees with his opinion or challenges him, he uses anger to punish her, to frighten her into seeing things his way, and make her change her behaviour. He believes that he has the *right* to use his anger to insist that she behaves the way he wants her to. It is a way of letting her know who is boss, of intimidating.

The result is that she uses every ounce of energy forever trying to be perfect in his eyes. If she believes a certain action of hers will anger him, she will avoid doing it – but, of course, all he will do is find another excuse for abusing her, however much he may show remorse or behave lovingly for long periods.

Sally told me that, though Guy never physically abused her, she dreaded his anger. 'However much you know he is unjustified,' she says, 'it is soul-destroying. You absorb it, you *do* begin to think, "Perhaps he is right, perhaps it is my fault." When someone is really shouting at you, and they are really, really angry, you just want to curl up and die. I found I would go out of my way to avoid upsetting him, I just couldn't bear his anger. I began to think, "I'm so bad, I've made him angry. Look what I've done." It made me feel guilty, worthless, absolutely exhausted by it all.'

For many abusive men, withholding attention and affection is as effective as shouting – sometimes more so. Often women tell me they would rather be shouted at than subjected to a silence in which they feel more frustrated, alone and helpless than ever.

One woman who came to Refuge was also deaf, and therefore already isolated. It was hard for her to communicate with anyone, let alone on such a sensitive subject, but she managed to tell me how her husband (a general practitioner, would you believe!) would deliberately hurt her by ignoring her. 'He would sulk for days if I did something he didn't like. I would be screaming for attention. I tried to shake him for attention and he just ignored me, sitting still. "Why can't you put your arms around me, why can't you?" I was begging. "I'm so frustrated, what about affection for me? I don't feel like you love me." He just wanted sex, that's all, not love.'

Some men, if they do not get their way, will maintain a wall of silence for days, ignoring every desperate attempt at communication or reconciliation on the part of a woman. They will come around when they are ready. Meanwhile their partners feel lonely and demeaned by their rejection.

Rebecca told me of her frustration when Ralph, instead of arguing a point, would frequently just withdraw. 'It was worse than anger,' she says. 'He would cut off, and I still see him now, walking upstairs with a cup of coffee in his hand to his own study, with the back of his neck *rigid* and a face like that, this is my vision of him. And he used to say, "I am self-controlled when we are having a row. I am controlled and I go away."'

Almost like a father controlling a child, Rebecca felt that Ralph was putting her in the position of forever having to try harder to gain his approval. He had the power to punish or reward her every word and action, and she never knew which it would be.

## 'No one understands about fear'

One of the most powerful ways in which abusive men control their partners is through fear. Even where no physical violence is involved, their unpredictable moods can instil fear into their partners.

However, many of the women I talk to are literally afraid for their lives, or for their children's lives, or they are afraid that, whatever they do or say, they will be subjected to more pain. People who have had no contact with women who live with violence find it hard to understand how they can stay in such a situation, but, as Melinda explains, 'They don't realise how trapped you are and how frightened you are.'

She recalls the moment when her husband Trevor, the man who had 'devastated' her with his charm, hit her for the first time. 'It was when the baby was crying in the night, and I got up to look after him,' she recalls. 'I was sitting cuddling him and Trevor came downstairs and told me to put him down and let him cry. I didn't want to and he slapped me.

'I didn't even really know about violence, that men hit women. If you read about it, you don't want to know about it – you forget it, shove it away. You don't think it will happen to you. I wasn't accustomed to being frightened by men. I wasn't accustomed to being frightened of anybody or anything before this. He terrified me. I felt really scared, and I felt that I'd got myself into something which I had no control over.'

Two years after Melinda summoned up the courage to leave Trevor, she confided to me, 'I'm still very frightened of him, and I will be until he's dead.'

I have seen women whose faces have been slashed with knives and battered with hammers. One woman who was attacked with a hammer and chisel had to have 250 stitches in her face. I will never forget her as long as I live – there was not an inch of untouched skin, just a mass of cuts and bruising. I had to feed her through a straw.

Other women have had boiling water poured over them, or suffered miscarriages because their husbands have hit them in the stomach while they are pregnant. Hazel had six miscarriages in all after her husband beat her. One man broke his wife's arm in three places and raped her three days after her baby was born, bursting her stitches.

Pregnancy is meant to be a time of happiness in a relationship, a time when a woman should feel cherished by her partner. Yet, ironically, pregnancy is a time when women are more vulnerable to violence. It is estimated that four to nine in every 100 pregnant women are abused during their pregnancy or soon after the birth.[10] Other research shows there is a link between abuse during pregnancy and a woman's chance of being killed by her perpetrator.[11] In Refuge's own services, more than 20 per cent of the women we supported last year were pregnant or had recently had a baby. One woman told me: 'The violence started when I got pregnant. We were arguing after we had missed a restaurant booking. Suddenly he hit me and threw me across the room. Throughout the pregnancy I had to explain away the bruises from his punches and kicks. He kneed me in the stomach, and pushed me down the stairs; I had to tell the midwife that I fell. I was constantly accused of being hysterical and harming the baby – he even told me to apologise to the midwife when I gave birth, because I had been "too hysterical". After my son was born, he would keep me up screaming at me through the night, and criticise my parenting – while never taking care of the baby.'

These women are paralysed by fear. Above all it is the unpredictable nature of the violence which is most terrifying and debilitating. Remember that the abuser changes his skin like a chameleon: one minute he is vile, the next caring, comforting and charming. Charm Syndrome Man may cry, beg forgiveness, or promise that the abuse will never happen again. He may even threaten suicide if his partner leaves him.

Laura remembers that, when James first began to be violent towards her, he appeared to be in agony over what he had done. 'He would beg me not to leave him,' she says. 'He'd say that I was the only one who could help him, the only one who understood. And if I left him, he wouldn't be able to go on. He said he'd make it better. He'd never, ever hurt me again... but of course he did.'

Melinda recalls, 'After that first time, when Trevor hit me, he seemed to be as shocked as I was. He kept saying: "My God, I didn't mean to do it. I don't know what happened to me." He seemed so distraught. I just wanted to make him feel better about it. Make it all right again.'

An abuser can be kind, considerate and loving for such long periods that the woman minimises the pain, even puts it out of her mind, or blames herself for causing it, vowing to be more careful in the future. But, as Laura found, after a period of calm, and without warning, some trivial incident would trigger the violence again. Gradually, the woman finds herself becoming more nervous, more wary, more afraid, never knowing how her partner is going to behave. Shot through the pattern of control is unpredictability.

Melinda told me that, as the abuse began to escalate, Trevor would go out with friends until three or four in the morning, while she lay awake 'terrified', never knowing whether or not he would decide to assault her when he came home. 'He would say, "What are you frightened about? I only beat you once a month."' Melinda recalls, 'At that time it *was* only once a month. And I'd say, "Because you could hit me *tonight*. It doesn't matter that it's only once a month, it might be tonight, and it's the waiting and the winding up that's the worst."'

For Melinda, like most women in this situation, one of the most terrifying things was that, after she had been hit once, she always lived in fear of it happening again. An abuser does not even have to strike again. Once he has instilled that fear, he has all the control. 'I couldn't win,' Melinda goes on. 'If he decided he wanted to beat me up, he would find anything… the soap would be on the right side of the taps instead of the left, that sort of thing. If I wasn't respectful enough… The two or three times I did stand up to him, I nearly got killed. I mean he would throttle me unconscious, so a lot of it was fear. When he told me he would kill me if I told anyone what he did to me, I had no reason to doubt him. He'd done such awful things.'

Hazel, too, ended up living in fear of Jimmy, unnerved above all by the unpredictability. Like so many abused women, she says, 'I used to hope that he would change, or that I could somehow change him – that hope went on for a long, long time. He had a belt, and he used to hit me with that, you know, the buckle, and he'd use it if I didn't get out of the room in time. And he'd keep a knife by the bed. Towards the end of the marriage, the abuse got more severe, and it got more frequent. I was demented, absolutely terrified. I just didn't know who to turn to. In fact I was thinking about suicide towards the end.'

Hazel had been to the police, to her priest and to social services – all of whom had failed to help her. The best offer she had received was to put her children into care – leaving her on the streets. She felt that she was left to handle her terror alone. Once, Jimmy tried to choke her, at the same time ramming his knee into her so hard that she later had to have surgery for a ruptured spleen. 'My head was buzzing, and my ears were popping, and the *fear*…his face was totally distorted,' says Hazel. 'I just wanted to close his eyes, I didn't want them to be the last thing I saw when I died. I went to close his eyes, but he thought I was going to claw him, and he got up and he went in the other room. Now he had kept his air rifle there, but I had hidden the pellets, so he couldn't shoot at me – he had tried that before. But he kept a pickaxe handle up there. He'd said it was there in case there was a burglar because there had been a lot of burglaries, and he came back with the pickaxe handle and he said, "Right, you're going to die this time."

'He went to swing with it and I put my hands up and grabbed it, but I wasn't strong enough to keep it off, and it went across my neck. I had a mark across my neck for about six months. I told him I would do anything he wanted if he'd let me loose. And as soon as I promised that I would do anything he wanted, he stopped and he went to the toilet, and he was ranting and raving so much that I crawled down the stairs and got out to the front door, and he never heard.

'It sounds strange, but what I wanted to do was to run underneath a hedge, curl up and die. I was so frightened. I didn't want to die violently, but just in my head I wanted to die. I was so blind, frightened with terror, I kept running towards the fields, I just wanted to hide under the hedge; that was all I could think of.'

Eventually, Hazel ran to a friend's house. She took her to Jimmy's sister, who called the police. But even then she was too frightened to bring charges.

An abuser can instil fear into his partner simply by threatening or hinting at it, sometimes in many subtle ways, such as driving recklessly or clasping his hands around her neck, swearing and shouting, cutting up her clothes, harming pets, pounding his fists on the table or slamming lids onto saucepans while she is cooking. One woman, whose husband never physically abused her, was nonetheless paralysed by fear through such methods. She told me: 'He once beat to death two pigeons in our garden, just because they were annoying him. Then he hung them up, bleeding, from the fence. It was chilling – like it was a warning.'

This is psychological abuse: a kind of mental torture which keeps the woman on edge, never knowing when her partner's threats and insinuations are for real.

Acts such as shouting or smashing possessions might not seem terrifying in themselves, but if the woman knows that at any time they could signal physical violence against herself or her children, that is a very different matter. She spends all her time avoiding the anger which frightens her so much. She is controlled by fear.

Melinda told me of a horrifying moment when Trevor, who was over six feet tall and weighed 17½ stone threatened her in the kitchen. 'He took a knife out of the drawer and held it against my throat,' she says. 'Then he waved it about and he said to me, "I'm going to stick this up your vagina and turn it around until there's nothing left." And I looked at his face and he was like some wild maniac. And I thought, "My God!" He didn't do it, but I believed he was capable of it.

'I think it was at that moment that I made up my mind that if he ever threatened me like that, or hit me again, I was getting out and that I was never ever going back, no matter what he said or did.'

Abusive men often play with 'weapons' in front of their partners to instil fear. Hazel's husband kept a knife by the bed. One man kept an axe under his pillow, threatening that if his wife ever tried to leave, he would use it. In the end, she was so terrified, she could not sleep at night for fear that if she so much as turned over in bed, her husband would lash out with the axe.

Laura's university-educated husband had beaten her so badly – on one occasion she miscarried after he hit her in the stomach and locked her out in the freezing cold – that even after they separated he could terrify her with phone calls threatening to harm both her and the children. One minute during these calls he would appear calm and rational, the next he would scream at her, 'Fucking bitch! I'm going to come and kill you all!'

'I mean, I had to go and get an alarm system put in,' she says, 'because I was so terrified that he would come round in the middle of the night over the roof, through the attic, or break in through the basement and come and kill us all. He threatened to do it, and I knew he was capable of it.'

Finally Laura taped some of his calls and played them back to me. What made them particularly chilling was the menace in James's voice. He would tell her, 'If you want a quiet life, do as I say, or else...' So powerful were the tapes that Laura played them to her solicitor before going to court, to convince him of the kind of abuse she was being subjected to. 'He had obviously heard all this kind of thing before, and it didn't really strike home,' says Laura. 'Then I said, "Look, please, please listen to these tapes", and he did listen to them and I could tell that they had swung it completely in his mind. He said, "Right, what you need is an injunction. I can tell the sort of man he is." It just made it seem real for him, rather than hearing another story about a domestic row where a wife had got hit.'

Charm Syndrome Man unashamedly uses the threat of violence to frighten his partner into staying with him. 'If you try to leave, I'll find you and kill you' is a typical threat. Hazel says, 'Jimmy had me totally convinced that he would kill me, and that nobody could save me. All throughout my marriage I was totally convinced – afterwards when I'd got out of it, I was still totally convinced that he would come after me one day.'

Frequently women like Hazel are frightened not only for themselves, but for family, friends or their children too – because Charm Syndrome Man frequently involves them in his threats. Often the women I talk to show tremendous courage in staying in intolerable situations, rather than put their families at risk.

Jimmy knew that if he involved the children when he became violent towards Hazel, he could always remain in control. 'The time he fired at me with his air rifle,' she says, 'Mark, my son, was in the kitchen. I hadn't got him out – you know when you run in blind panic – and he was screaming, so I couldn't run away, and I couldn't run back while Jimmy was firing. So I waited until he ran out of pellets, then I ran across to get Mark, and Jimmy went and gave me a good hiding, and just kept Mark because he knew I couldn't get away because he had the bairn. Whenever he had the children, he knew he had me because I wouldn't leave the children.'

Another woman who phoned me in desperation echoed the terror many women feel in this situation. After a particularly vicious attack, sparked off by her having cooked something her husband did not like for dinner, she could not take any more of his violence. She had gone upstairs to throw a few things into a bag, and the next thing she knew she was being thrown over her daughter's bed and flung down the stairs. Her husband told her that *she* could leave but not the children – and the catch was if she did go, the children would be dead when she got back. So obviously she stayed.

Three days after this, during which time she says she shook with fear, her husband agreed to leave. 'It was all sorted out. Everything was going okay,' she said. 'He'd moved out and I was happy, and then he turned up out of the blue. He was on his "I love you, I need you" routine, and asked to come back. I said no because I had no regrets over what I had done at all. He didn't get violent this time, but his temper was so bad that I could hardly move with fear.'

At the time she rang me, she and her husband were still living apart, but he constantly turned up threatening her. 'I'm frightened to go for a custody or restriction order,' she told me. 'As once he finds out, he'll smash my door down, kill me and take the kids, and they'd go through a living hell if he had them.'

However paradoxical it may appear, women in this situation often feel less frightened staying with their abusers than if they leave them. At least, they tell me, they have some idea of where they are. They feel they have some element of control over their situation. For example, in one of the most sickening cases of violence I have encountered, one woman whose face was scarred from knife attacks, came to me after being so brutally attacked that her skull had been exposed. Although she had actually run away from her live-in boyfriend, she confessed that it was almost a relief when he tracked her down. The subsequent beating she suffered was less terrifying than never knowing when he might pounce down a dark alley, or break down the door in the middle of the night.

Knowing that there is someone out there with one thing on his mind – to kill you or beat you – is one of the most frightening things any woman can go through. Women tell me that it dominates everything: they cannot think about anything else, only the idea of being tracked down and hurt again. Even when they have ceased to live with them, such men are still able to control their partners mercilessly.

Often the threat of violence is directed at other targets close to the woman, such as family pets or personal possessions. Hazel said that Jimmy 'told me he would get me and I felt he would – it was a definite threat – because he had no compulsion about killing anything. I mean he would kill an animal. I had a dog called Raffles and he shot her in the head. He'd been out with her and a younger dog, and Raffles came home before him, and when he came home he shot her in front of me and the boys. Because she defied him by coming home early.' If a man kills a pet, what is to stop him from killing his wife?

Trevor alternated between threatening Melinda and taking out his anger on her possessions. This may seem less frightening than a physical attack, but the abuser is in fact being very selective in his violence. He is in control. He will not smash anything that will affect his own enjoyment, he will never demolish his own possessions. His violence is centred on his partner and, by destroying the things she loves, he hurts and frightens her by implying that she could easily be the next target.

Melinda says, 'The place that we lived in when we first married was my flat in my name, and every stick of furniture was mine, so he used to take pleasure in destroying everything that was mine, that I'd spent so long in getting together. He used to throw my glasses across the room and break them, and punch the pictures and that sort of thing – punch the walls, put his fist through the wall – never,' she notes, 'the television or anything like that.'

Another woman I talked to told a similar story. On one occasion, she revealed, after she had returned home slightly later than expected from visiting her sick mother, she found 'all my clothes taken out of the wardrobe, and ripped up on the floor – everything'. Many women tell me their partners have ripped or cut up their clothes, and they find it a particularly humiliating form of abuse. One woman told how her husband would rip her clothes with a Stanley knife, while she was actually wearing them.

It is impossible to underestimate the effects that fear, bound up as it is with intense emotions, can have on a woman – especially when the situation is confused by the fact that, however frightening these men can be, this is only one facet of their characters. They are perfectly capable of reverting to being charming, kind and sometimes full of remorse. Sometimes they do not even need to be charming: just a period of being calm and 'normal' seems like bliss to a woman who has just suffered horrifying abuse.

Melinda is well aware that, while she stayed with her husband, her fear was tied up with bewilderment, because he was able to switch to love and affection so easily. 'He confused me,' she explains. 'He got round me so successfully with his utter contrition. I felt trapped, very trapped by everything.'

Frequently, when abused women talk to me over a period of time, there are days when I have to remind them of the horrors they have previously recounted, because in the period after the violence their husbands and partners have been kind and loving, and the bad times seem temporarily a thing of the past.

Melinda, like most of the women who contact Refuge, knew only too well how hard it was to try to explain this to people. She had almost lost her job twice, because she was so badly beaten that she repeatedly failed to turn up for work. Though her husband had warned her, 'If you tell anybody what I do to you, I'll kill you', when her job was threatened for the second time, she did try to explain to her bosses what was happening. But she found, 'In the end, people got fed up with me, because they didn't know how difficult it is to get away. They couldn't understand. They'd just say, "Just tell him to go. He's horrible." And they think you're not strong enough. I think they thought I was silly.

'They don't realise about fear.'

## 'The bedroom was a battleground'

For many women sexual abuse is often the hardest of all to bear, because it violates such an intimate area of their lives. They feel defiled and humiliated, and it is often hard for them to talk about their experiences. When a woman is in bed with her partner she is often at her most vulnerable. If he violates their sense of closeness and trust, she feels attacked at the most intimate level.

Laura, like most of the women I talk to, found it desperately difficult to erase from her mind images of the sexual abuse that James had inflicted on her. At least, she told me: 'Physical abuse is sort of clean, if you know what I mean. Sexual abuse is so personal and so much the opposite of what it's meant to be, I suppose. There you are, two people together, and you're supposed to be gentle and loving to each other, and you have the exact opposite going on.'

In a loving relationship the sexual act is a shared thing, an expression of love and togetherness. In an abusive situation, the sexual act is about power. It is about a man's control over a woman. He may use it to show her who is boss, to punish her or to show his contempt for her. One woman told me: 'My husband would tell me that making love to me was like going to the toilet. He only did it to relieve himself. So can you imagine that in the back of your head? All the time he is making love he is only doing it to relieve himself!'

Sexual abuse can take many forms. It can involve physical, emotional, psychological and verbal pain, often all bound up together. A man may force a woman to take part in acts which she finds degrading and offensive, such as anal sex or group sex or even sex in front of the children.

He may threaten violence if she refuses sex – Lisa, the deaf woman, says, 'You had to do it, or you got hit.' Or he may insist on sex *after* violence – like Beverley's husband, Dave. 'I could never understand it,' she says. 'There's nothing sexual about violence. It certainly doesn't turn me on, it petrifies me. And that's the last thing I'd want to do when he'd had a go at me.'

Many men actually wound their partners during sexual acts. I have even known women who have had bottles forced into their vaginas. Laura told me: 'James would hit me while we were supposedly making love, or he'd say, "I demand my rights" and hit me, and I would say, "This is not the way to go about things", and he'd say, "Yes it is, and you're going to smile while you're doing it." And I think I found that the hardest to cope with, and also the most long-term thing to get over.

'The first time it happened he came into the room when I was dead asleep. My daughter was in bed with me, because I was still breastfeeding her. James dragged me out of bed by my hair across to the spare room, threw me across the bed, and shoved his penis in my mouth. And I'd been dead asleep, and suddenly to be dragged across the room like this, and thrown on the bed...I just bit as hard as I could.

'I thought, "Jesus, he's going to kill me now" because, you know, I'd done it instinctively, and you do such stupid things. I put the light on because I'd thought he's not going to kill me if he can see me, so I put the electric light on and I was absolutely terrified. Obviously he didn't kill me – he just roared and shouted at me and said, "Don't you ever bite me again", and I quaked and shook.

'When I think about it now, I think, "Why the hell didn't I just walk out?" I know people will think I was crazy to stay – but I had nowhere to go, no job. And there was the baby. The way he treated me made me feel so dirty and worthless as well. I suppose you could say I felt exploited. Anyway, I just couldn't think how I could begin to tell anybody. Who would understand?

'The other thing was – and I know it's hard to believe – in between the horrible bits, he'd have phases when he was so gentle and loving, that I'd put them to the back of my mind. But eventually it got to the stage where I was terrified of having sex with him, because I didn't know how it was going to be.

'Eventually, I burst into tears in front of my aunt, who made me tell her what was wrong, and it all came out. She was so horrified she said, "Right, you're leaving now", and I did – but without her financial support I doubt if I could have managed. My aunt is a wealthy woman, so she was able to find me somewhere to live, and she bought me a car, so that I could get my independence back.

'It wasn't just the money, though. Emotionally I was in such a state, I literally couldn't think what to do next. By that stage, I could barely even decide how much milk to order in the mornings, let alone what I was going to do with the rest of my life.'

Hazel's husband combined violent sexual abuse with verbal abuse, calling her filthy names, which she could not bear. 'That abused me mentally, the filthy language. And because I had been sexually abused, the filthy language seemed to fit, do you know what I mean? If it fits, you believe it.'

Often men use verbal abuse to degrade a woman when it comes to sex: telling their partners they are frigid, that they are useless in bed or suggesting that they are lesbians. One woman confided, 'There was a little girl, she was about ten, who used to come around because she used to play with my son, who was 11. But my husband used to say, "Why is she here? Are you a lesbian?" It was just an excuse to start on me again. So in the end I couldn't have anybody to the house.'

Many women do not actually know that they are being sexually abused, because they bear no scars, and their partners have never forced them to do anything they found degrading. When I asked one woman if her husband had ever sexually abused her, she replied, 'No, not really... except when I was off the pill for one month between one pill and another, and because I wouldn't favour him when I was off the pill, he thought, "Well, you're my wife, and you'll do as I say", and that was it.' Like many women, she was expected to have sex with her husband as and when he wanted it. That is a form of sexual abuse. *She* is not in control over what happens to her body – *he* is. When a woman lives with an abusive man, he controls their sex life. They have sex when he wants to, without any consideration for her feelings.

Some abusers prevent women from using contraception as a method of control. Hazel's husband, Jimmy, threatened to kill her if she ever left him. 'You'll never be free of me,' he vowed. She says, 'He was always trying to get me pregnant. I mean, he thought it was really great when, a year after Mark was born, I got pregnant with twins [which she subsequently lost]. He was always forcing himself upon me when I wasn't using any contraception. It was like a sort of game or a battle, really. If I used a contraceptive cap, he used to take it out and throw it across the room. And there's me frantically counting up days in my head, wondering if I was okay or not.' One woman described how, looking back, making her pregnant was one way her husband increased her dependency and isolation. 'It was his way of keeping me the "little missus" at home,' she said.

It is very easy for people to ask, 'Why doesn't she just say no?' But as Sally says, 'The times I did say no, there would be hysterics. He'd accuse me either of being frigid, not caring, or having an affair with someone else. In the end giving in was the easier option. But it made me feel as though I had no control over my body. I was just an object, to be used, as and when he liked. I'd never felt that way before. I don't think I thought of it as "sexual abuse" – I just knew that I felt bad about it. I had never thought a man could ever make me feel that way, which was even more disturbing.'

Melinda, too, was unaware that she had suffered sexual abuse, yet she told me: 'After Emma had been born – that's my youngest – I'd had a Caesarean, I'd nearly died, I'd been desperately ill and when I came home from hospital he insisted on making love to me the morning I got back. And I was in terrible pain. *Nothing* was further from my mind, and he just insisted.'

Laura told me that towards the end of her marriage James demanded sex without any regard for her feelings. 'I remember,' she says, 'that he demanded sex after my second child was born. It was far too soon and far too brutal, and in a way I knew it was a test. It wasn't nice at all.' She was hurt and angered by this incident, but she had learned to bottle up her anger; she was worn out after the birth of her baby, terrified of James's reaction, and she so much wanted a peaceful, happy home for the new baby that she gave in to James's demands.

One woman was suffering from pneumonia and toxaemia after having her first baby. Her husband did not even bother to come and visit her in hospital, yet as soon as she came home he forced her to have sex. She had had 17 stitches, which broke. 'I was too ashamed and frightened to go back to the hospital,' she told me. 'I couldn't have stopped him, but I thought they would tell me off.'

It was only in 1991 that rape within marriage became illegal. Yet many men still think they have the right to force a woman to have sex against her will in her own home. An Englishman's home is his castle: apparently he can do what he likes behind his own closed doors.

Unfortunately, our society still endorses that view: women are still brought up to believe they should be ready and willing to satisfy their partner's every sexual need as part of their wifely duties (and that often includes things they find distasteful). And abusive men insist on their 'conjugal rights' without ever stopping to consider that their partners might like a say in the matter.

I say, what about an English*woman*'s home being *her* castle? A woman should be able to say no. She should never have to give in to sex simply because she is scared to refuse, or because it is her only way of preventing a row – otherwise it is rape.

Looking back, Hazel is in no doubt about what was happening to her. 'I was being used. I mean, they say you can't be raped in marriage, but you can.' She recalls one night when Jimmy forced himself on her. Incredible as it may seem today, he insisted, 'I am your husband and you have to give it to me. You can't refuse your husband. It is my right to have sex with you.'

'He jumped on top of me,' says Hazel, 'and I said "Uh" and shut my eyes, thought of England – thought of anything, but I was fighting him, because I didn't want him near me. At that stage he was really punching me, holding my arms down on the bed. He was raping me. There was a knock on the door. It was so lucky. I pulled him off and said, "Look, it might be my dad", and he just went really quiet and something snapped in his head and he stopped. I jumped off that bed, threw my trousers and jumper on and I just flew out of that flat. I don't think anybody can believe how you can be abused. Eventually I just couldn't take it anymore.'

Paradoxically, women often do not want to say no to sex, even though they are not really in the mood, because they hope that the sexual act might revive the loving, caring side of their partners, the side they fell in love with – the charming side. Even if they have no choice in the matter, this may be the only area which offers a brief respite from the physical and emotional abuse which colours the rest of their relationship.

Sometimes, because a couple's sexual relationship remains good, a woman blinds herself to the realities of what is happening in other areas. She is confused: how could he make love to her so passionately if he did not really care for her? That is exactly the argument Charm Syndrome Man uses. If she threatens to leave, he will say, 'How can you doubt the way I feel – look how good our sex life is.' Even after the most violent rows, he will try to control his partner by making love to her tenderly and lovingly, encouraging her to forgive and forget his bad behaviour.

'Ralph seemed to think that all he had to do, after he had been really angry and abusive, was sweep me off to bed and make love to me – and it would be all okay in the morning. No further discussion required,' says Rebecca. 'That was the last thing I wanted to do. I wanted to talk things through, and make friends properly. I always felt cheated. I never had a chance to have my say – it was just assumed that all I needed was sex. That was his answer to everything.'

Just as an abusive man uses sex as and when he wants it, he can humiliate and wound his partner's feelings by *refusing* to make love to her. In a healthy relationship one partner might be too tired to make love, or simply not in the mood, yet there are ways of saying no, without hurting the other's feelings. An abuser, on the other hand, will tell his partner she is frigid, ugly and undesirable, that she does not satisfy him or that he should never have married her. If *he* has sexual problems, he will blame them on her. Or he may put her down, calling her a slut for making the first move, leaving her feeling guilty, confused and rejected.

Often an abusive man backs up this rejection of his partner in bed by ogling other women in front of her, and making unfavourable comparisons when they are out together. She feels humiliated, and her self-confidence fades, so that even when he is loving and gentle again, she finds it very hard to respond.

While such battles are going on in the bedroom, abusive men are frequently also being unfaithful – though such behaviour would be unthinkable in their partners. One man sexually abused his wife a few weeks before he left her for another woman. 'I thought he was going to make love to me in the normal way,' she says, 'and I partly reacted, but then he started being violent and then he threw me on the bed and attacked me from behind and he penetrated me from behind – it was terrible. He was a big man and his weight on me hurt my left hip, and it was many months before the strain was relieved, I had to have treatment from an osteopath for it. So that was absolutely disgusting. He said because he was in love with this woman, he couldn't have sex with me in the normal way, because it would be adultery, and only with this woman he loved was it normal.'

This man was humiliating and degrading his wife in a very calculated way in order to remind her who was in control. The more ashamed and demeaned she felt, the more superior he felt, and the more he was able to dominate her.

Many men continue to behave in this way, even after they have separated from their partners. Women frequently tell me that their husbands and boyfriends come back, under the pretence of collecting belongings or seeing the children, and then rape them – as if they still have to prove that they have the upper hand.

## 'He controlled the purse strings'

An abusive man will try to control the purse strings, just as he tries to control every area of his partner's life. Taking a woman's wages or benefits, preventing her from getting or keeping a job, running up debts in her name or even withholding money so that she can barely afford to buy her children nappies are all things that can form part of an abuser's pattern of control, alongside psychological and physical abuse. Research by Refuge and The Co-operative Bank found that 18 per cent of all UK adults had experienced financial abuse in their relationships – and that 60 per cent of victims were women. Women rarely experience financial abuse in isolation – 86 per cent said they also experienced other forms of abuse.[12]

An abusive man uses the giving or withholding of money as a symbol of his power over his partner. If their income is low and she is unable to work because they have children, he will constantly remind her that she cannot survive without him. Not only does that idea reinforce his control over her, but it often prevents her from leaving.

Even women from comfortable backgrounds can be trapped in the same way. It is a myth to assume that such women have their own resources or easy access to joint funds. Many women who live with abusive men have to ask their partners every time they want to make a purchase, often having to submit minute details so that a decision can be made about whether or not they are *allowed* to have a new coat or a pair of shoes. I have known abusive men to stop paying their share of the mortgage, or the school fees. Or, post-separation, refusing to give their former partners any money at all to support themselves and their children.

Even if a woman has an independent career, it is not unusual for an abusive man to manipulate her into a situation where he is in control of their finances. Or he is so extravagant that she has to bail him out of financial trouble. She is often dependent on his 'generosity' for every penny she has for herself, the children or the housekeeping. One woman I supported, whose husband was very wealthy, was only given a paltry sum to spend on everything – including food and all the things their baby daughter needed. Yet he would get angry if there were not lavish meals cooked for him in the evening. This woman ended up buying the expensive food her husband wanted but asked the cashier to put some of it on her overdraft so the amount taken out of the joint account did not exceed the limit her husband imposed. And even in less extreme situations, if a woman looks carefully at her life, she usually realises that *he* makes the decisions about how and when to spend money, even if she is the breadwinner. Not only is he controlling the financial aspect of their relationship, he is also tying her to him more irrevocably. If she is dependent on him for money, it is so much harder for her to leave.

Sally happily used her student loan to buy king prawns and fillet steak to satisfy Guy's love of good food; she even delved into her loan money to buy petrol for his car. Yet, she recalls, 'On one occasion he got hysterical because I asked him for some money to buy tampons. By this time my student loan had almost run out. I didn't think it was unreasonable to ask for a box of tampons out of his money. At the time I was really furious, but he was so busy ranting and raving I didn't get a word in edgeways. Eventually I let the whole thing blow over.

'Another time when I had finished studying and was working, we were on holiday with friends in Scotland and I bought my niece a very inexpensive woolly hat – it was a real bargain. He rowed about this for three days in front of our friends, even over the dinner table. He maintained *we* couldn't afford it (even though I had my own income and bank account!) and put me down for being frivolous. Privately, my friends said they couldn't believe his reaction.'

Many abused women tell me that their husband or boyfriend spends all their money on himself, leaving his partner struggling to buy things for herself and their children. One woman told me: 'My husband was getting a cooked meal at work every day, but he wasn't giving me enough money to buy food at home. Some weeks I just had my child benefit, so I'd be buying potatoes and bread and nappies and things like that...just eating lots of chips and bread.'

Like Sally, this woman was also humiliated when she asked for money to buy tampons. 'He wanted to know how much they were, and when I came back he held his hand out for the penny change! He said, "It's *my* change – I want it."'

Jimmy's money went on drinking and smoking and gambling, yet Hazel felt guilty about complaining, because he frequently turned the tables on her, reverting to the man who 'could charm the birds out of the trees', spending extravagantly on her, buying her a new jacket, a handbag or perfume.

Charm Syndrome Man is frequently careless with money – he will insist on romantic weekends away, or expensive meals, even though he and his partner are broke. Then he will blame her for the fact that they have no money, and expect her to bail him out of trouble.

One woman, in her sixties, who had been subjected to emotional and sometimes violent abuse for years, told me her husband was 'very childish with money. In the end I was the manager and ran the bank accounts.' She was the main earner, but that did not stop him from feeling he had every right to spend all her money. 'When I first met him,' she says, 'he had nothing. He didn't even have a car, so I had put more into the marriage financially than he had. I also earned more than he did. When he was out of work for two years, it didn't even occur to me to think that I was keeping him; it was just one of those things.

'When I was 55, I was offered early retirement – you get a lump sum and one-third of your salary as a pension – I'd thought about it and I didn't really want to give up work, but I remember him looking at the pension details and saying, "*We* will get this lump sum, *we* will never get the chance to get our hands on a lump sum like that again. We'll invest it." The more he talked about it, the more I thought, "Well, why not?" So I took early retirement the following September. The day after I put the money in our joint account, he bought a new top-of-the-range car.'

Shortly afterwards, this woman's husband abandoned her for another woman, sexually assaulting her before he went. 'When he left home he took what remained in the account,' she says. 'He said, "It was out of the joint account, therefore it was mine." I was left with nothing. He also took the car, leaving me with his battered wreck, which I've still got.' She had had no idea that her husband was seeing another woman, and despite the fact that he often slapped her and regularly put her down, she loved him, trusted him and was totally committed to their future together. The last thing that had entered her head when she was making her financial arrangements was that he might empty their bank account and leave her. His behaviour left her both financially and emotionally shattered. Later, to twist the knife even further, he deliberately became unemployed so that he could not be made to support his wife. Even when he abandoned her, he was still exercising control.

Indeed, financial abuse can be one of the most enduring forms of abuse, its effects lasting long after a woman has left. One woman came to Refuge with £20,000 worth of credit card debt after her boyfriend coerced her into paying his bills and handing over her wages. She had to borrow money from family members in order to live, which affected the whole family's finances for years to come.

An abuser might demand that a woman hands over her hard-earned wages, but it is just as common for him to prevent her from working. Of course, in many families where the men work while the women take on the lion's share of the childcare, the women are perfectly happy because this is a choice they have made. Their husbands and partners are generous and open about financial matters, and the women do not feel frightened to ask for their share. However, for an abuser, forcing a woman to stay at home is a way of reducing her escape routes and breaking down her sense of self. One woman, who was forced to give up the job she loved by her violent ex-husband, put it like this: 'Work was a big part of my identity. It wasn't just about financial independence; work gave me a bigger pool to swim in. It meant I was mixing with "outsiders" who might have pricked my consciousness. They might have made me think, "What's happening to me isn't right."'

## 'I must be to blame'

Charm Syndrome Man puts his own interpretation on events, twisting the emphasis so that his partner is to blame for his abusive behaviour.

'Jimmy blamed me for everything – it was always my fault,' says Hazel. 'He said I provoked him. If I hadn't argued with him, nagged him or upset him or whatever you want to call it, then I wouldn't have been hit. He always twisted it around afterwards so that I ended up comforting *him*, to make him feel better for what he'd done.'

Hazel suspected Jimmy was having affairs. 'But', she says, 'if I asked him about it, he told me I had a wicked mind. After a while you think you *must* have a wicked mind, you know. Everything was my fault. I mean it was my fault because I answered back, it was my fault he couldn't find his cigarettes, and if the shops were closed it was my fault. I mean I used to go around apologising.'

The abused women I talk to almost always feel guilty and ashamed. They feel that they have failed in their relationships, that they must have in some way caused their partner's abusive behaviour: 'If I hadn't done this, if only I had kept quiet, if only, if only...' One woman whose husband had abused her for 15 years – he frequently held knives to her throat and threatened her with his gun – said to me, a whole ten years after she had escaped to a remote Scottish island, 'Actually, I think I was partly to blame.'

Hazel was tortured by such feelings: 'I was frightened for a long time that it was something in me that attracted this in him. I thought I brought it out in him. Even after I left him, I would be feeling guilty. Now I've realised that it wasn't me at all – because friends have told me he behaves even more badly with his second wife.'

When Melinda first contacted me, one of the first questions she asked was: 'What part do I play in the abuse?' Trevor had convinced her that she was to blame for his behaviour. 'I think what kept me very confused,' she says, 'was the guilt. I thought it was all my fault. That is what Trevor used to tell me. He'd say he never had arguments with anyone else.

'There was a whole period of time in which he had told me that it was my fault, that it was my behaviour that caused his violence towards me. If I had had a couple of glasses of wine with dinner and he was abusive later, he would say I was drunk and had provoked him. He said our friends didn't like coming around anymore because I was irritable – I'm sure I was on occasions, but is it any wonder when I was living on tenterhooks all the time, not knowing how he would behave?

'And because I was cut off from myself, I was cut off from the outside world, I was cut off from all my friends – anybody who knew what was going on in that relationship – I suppose the only logic seemed to be to believe it *was* all my fault.' If only she could change or stop provoking him, she believed, the abuse would stop too. As she says, 'If Trevor was telling me it was *my* fault, and making me believe that, then, if it was *my* fault, I could also make it better.'

Because women like Melinda are so isolated, they are frequently unsure of themselves. There is no one to tell them that they are not to blame. All sources of support are barred to them. 'The crazy thing,' says Melinda, 'is that Trevor was the one who would comfort me after the abuse. He would tell me how lucky I was to have someone as caring and understanding as him to look after me, which only made me feel guilty for having wanted to leave.

'I used to search and search and search for what I had done wrong that caused the dreadful abuse. It must be my fault, it must be something I had done, how could I change it? That idea that it was my fault became the cornerstone of the relationship – and it was only when I was able to talk to people who made me see that I wasn't to blame that I began to build my self-esteem and confidence and get out of the very tight web of that relationship.'

Hazel took her guilt one stage further: 'I blamed myself for marrying him,' she says. 'I felt it was my own fault. I blamed myself all the time. I carried the burden of this guilt and shame around with me. But now I realise I didn't deserve to be treated like that and nobody does. No human being deserves to be treated like that. But there are a lot of women still trapped by guilt.'

# 'Think of the children'

Many abusers involve the children, to make their partners feel even more guilty. One woman told me that her daughter came to her and said, 'Couldn't you try to be nicer to Daddy?' He had completely poisoned the children against me,' the woman told me. 'He told them that the rows were all my fault. That he didn't know what to do. He'd tried, but I was impossible...Can you imagine how I felt? Frustrated, hurt, angry and guilty.'

It is not unusual for an abuser to tell the children, without foundation, that their mother drinks too much, or does not look after him properly – leaving the woman feeling she is to blame not just for the abuse, but for tension in the house. If he behaves badly in front of the children, she frequently feels guilty for not protecting them from such scenes.

Not only do abused women feel guilty within their relationships, but it is often guilt which prevents them from leaving. They believe that it is wrong to abandon their partners and split up their families, however bad their situation is. Still, society bombards women with messages that they should get a man – and keep him – at all costs, putting him and their relationship first; she should make sacrifices and take the rough with the smooth. Women feel guilty about putting themselves first.

On the contrary, focusing on her own needs can be the best thing for a woman's children. Staying for the sake of the children keeps her trapped unnecessarily – women think they are doing the right thing, believing that they can shield the children from the violence and keep the family together. Children are almost always aware that violence is occurring at home. Often, the last straw will be when the man starts hitting the children.

Sixty-two per cent of children living in domestic abuse households are directly harmed by the perpetrator of the abuse – but for the remaining 38 per cent, the impacts can still be severe.[13] One in five children have been exposed to domestic abuse.[14] One Canadian study found that as many as three to five children in every classroom could be exposed to domestic violence at home.[15] An estimated 39,000 babies are thought to be living with domestic violence in the UK.[16] In the same way that non-physical abuse can be just as harmful to women as physical abuse, exposure to traumatic events – including witnessing domestic violence at home – can affect children profoundly. Impacts can be physical, emotional and behavioural. Children can experience profound fear and distress, and even develop post-traumatic stress disorder, experiencing nightmares or flashbacks, hypervigilance and difficulty in concentrating. Some show physical signs, such as bed-wetting or constant colds, mouth ulcers, asthma or eczema. Some children may become withdrawn and find it difficult to communicate, or they become anxious and clingy and experience low self-esteem or even depression. Often, they think they are to blame for the abuse and that it is their job to protect their mother or siblings. They may find it difficult to concentrate at school or regress developmentally. Older children are more likely to truant from school or take risks with alcohol and drugs.

Women living with abusive men are fighting for their basic survival while doing their best to attend to their children's needs – quite understandably, some may be less able to offer emotional support to their children, compounding these issues. Ground down by years of abuse, some women become depressed and emotionally detached from their children. Often, the perpetrator's power and control tactics target and undermine the mother's relationship with her child. Children regularly witness their father denigrating their mother; is it any wonder women sometimes feel they have little authority over their children? In turn, a role reversal may occur, with the child adopting a parenting role. Isolated from the support of family and friends, some mothers may treat their children as confidants – not realising how confusing this may be for their sons or daughters, as the parent they have relied on becomes increasingly reliant on them.[17]

It is important for a woman to know that children can overcome the impact of domestic violence with appropriate support and go on to live safe and happy lives. Children can develop their sense of self-worth through friends or other family members, or through achieving at school. Of course, many women feel guilty for underestimating or minimising the impact of abuse on their children – but doing so is understandable and very typical. Mothers often underestimate the extent to which their children witness or are affected by domestic violence.[18] One woman, who was violently abused by the father of her three children for more than a decade, told me: 'After I left, I used to feel so guilty for what my kids went through. I thought I was protecting them from it, but my son sometimes tells me things he remembers from when he was small and I realise I was kidding myself. I don't feel guilty anymore – I know I did the right thing and now we have a peaceful, happy life. I am a good mother who removed my family from a very difficult situation – I think when they're older, my kids will be proud of me for that. I am proud of myself.'

Women often tell me that they don't feel their personal happiness and fulfilment are good enough reasons to leave – that he isn't hitting the children, so it is better to keep the family together. The realisation that children are affected by living in an emotional war zone, even if they are not physically abused, can be a catalyst for leaving. A woman need not stay for their benefit. A violent father is not a positive role model – and as the catalogue of possible repercussions for children shows, living with violence and abuse takes its toll.

The experience of one woman I supported, Andrea, shows how children can be used as pawns by abusers not only while the relationship continues, but also afterwards. Andrea first met Felix at university as postgraduate students. He was intelligent, dynamic and gregarious. She recalls, 'He seemed so perfect – he liked everything that I liked. I thought he was my saviour. I had split up with my last boyfriend because he wasn't at all into family, but Felix was – he seemed really family-oriented, and I loved that.' They got together at a party, and Felix moved into Andrea's flat a few months later. 'It was quite a whirlwind.'

For the first two years, Andrea was happy – but then Felix's frequent bad moods worsened, to the point where he would regularly ignore her and their daughter, Millie. 'That is what is really tough,' Andrea says. 'Going from thinking "Well, I've just married someone who gets very grumpy and miserable – what can I do to cheer him up?" to realising that there is nothing you can do, to realising that the anger and vile behaviour, the name-calling and the stonewalling is not normal, it is abusive.'

Felix frequently used Millie to punish his wife. 'As Millie got older, I used to read to her every evening. Millie loved it, but he would stomp around the house slamming doors and playing loud music. Or he would actually come and stand next to us and roll his eyes and sigh. He would tell me Millie hated my reading, and that I should see her rolling her eyes at me with him.'

Felix could not stand for Andrea and Millie to have such shared moments without him, even though he was always asked to join in. He was jealous. Yet when Andrea encouraged him to spend time with his daughter, Millie often ended up crying. Andrea says, 'He just had no patience. I remember him sitting with her doing her homework and he would just get nastier and nastier, until she would burst into tears.

'Millie was once really unwell and I told him that she couldn't possibly go to school. I thought he would just say it was fine, but instead he made a massive point of undermining me and insisted that she was okay. It turned into the most horrific situation; he was so cross. That's when you start to feel destabilised – you're not saying anything controversial and yet the reaction is totally disproportionate.'

Andrea told me that during their separation – when they were still living under the same roof – Felix's behaviour towards Millie changed. All of the things he had been so dismissive of before, like reading to her, now had to be his domain. 'He made me feel like a ghost in my own home,' she said. 'Although I had been Millie's main carer since she was born, he suddenly wouldn't let me have anything to do with her. He would insist on taking her to school and picking her up; she should sit on the sofa with him, not me. Before I had a chance to say goodnight in the evenings, he would put her to bed, turn the light off and shut the door. I would have to sneak into her room in the dark to give her a kiss. Millie definitely picked up on it – sometimes she would rush over and give me a hug and say, "I'm sorry, Mummy."'

As far as Felix was concerned, only his happiness counted. Abusive men often use children as 'emotional property' – demonstrations of love and affection for children are a means of undermining and excluding their partners. Felix saw his opportunity to control Andrea emotionally through their daughter, and took it.

When I first met Andrea, she frequently said of Felix's behaviour, 'It sounds so silly now.' Of course, an outsider might hear of a man's bad mood and write it off as the ups and downs of any relationship – they might say Andrea shouldn't be so sensitive. But using children as weapons is part and parcel of a pattern of control.

Ralph frequently told Rebecca of her 'duty'. She said, 'He would tell me that if I left I would have failed, that there was something wrong with me if I couldn't cope with a little bit of anger, that it was all part of the rough and tumble of family life, and that I should see it in that context.' Had this been a 'normal' family life, with 'normal' ups and downs, Ralph might have had a point – no marriage runs smoothly all the time – but when a woman lives with an abuser, the downs are not in the least 'normal'. They are destructive and demoralising – and children absorb those feelings.

However, Rebecca wanted the marriage to work. She says, 'I tried to have that attitude as well. I could still look at him and see what a nice person he was, what a caring, loving, tender person he was, and what a good father he was to my children and I wanted to make all that work. I felt it should be my responsibility.' Bewitched by the charm, she felt she was to blame for the abuse. Ralph's control was complete.

## Abuse post-separation

If a woman is able to leave her perpetrator, he will often find any way he can to maintain a hold over her. For a man who is used to getting his way, 'his woman' leaving is a threat to his machismo, to the power he believes he is entitled to have. For men who have children with their victims, child contact arrangements provide ample opportunity to maintain control over their ex-partner. Such arrangements can also place children in difficult, if not frightening, situations. Some are asked to 'spy' on mothers, or provide information about any new relationships, and are threatened with abuse themselves if they do not comply. Young children often worry about inadvertently revealing their new address and become anxious as a result.

Even the family court itself – a state-sanctioned setting in which a woman should be able to feel safe – becomes a forum for abuse and intimidation. Family court rooms are often tiny, forcing the woman to sit close to the man who has abused her. There are rarely separate entrances or any form of special measures – such as the screens sometimes present in a criminal court – to lessen the trauma of coming face to face with her perpetrator. A man is able to bring repeated and often spurious court applications for child contact, subjecting his ex-partner to years of further anxiety and control, as well as financial abuse.

Practices that would never be allowed in criminal courts are commonplace in the family court. Hearings are conducted in private and – due to cuts in legal aid – women and their abusers are often left to represent themselves. There are many committed and sympathetic family lawyers working hard to support their clients – but not enough women can access them. Far too often in the family courts, the unthinkable happens; women are cross-examined by their abusers.

One woman who was supported by Refuge, Diana, was repeatedly abused by her perpetrator in the family court. When her ex-husband pursued access to their children, Diana found herself sitting in the same small court room as the man who had violently abused her for years. To begin with, both she and her ex had a barrister. The court's 'Fact Finding Hearing', which decides whether alleged incidents – in this case, of domestic violence – did or did not happen, found in Diana's favour on every count. But her abuser did not give up – and the cost of the proceedings so far meant Diana could no longer afford legal representation.

Over the next 24 months, Diana's perpetrator cross-examined her several times. She told me: 'I can barely put into words the terror I felt when my ex-husband questioned me directly in the family court. Fear stinks, and I know just how much. At the end of each "interrogation" I'd hide in the toilets and shake and sob, dousing myself in soap, water and perfume, trying desperately to wash away the experience.

'My ex taunted me about his violent past, name-calling and abusing me all over again. It happened on several occasions over many months. Each time was like being tortured. The officials whose protection I had sought watched impassively. Forcing me to relive the horror of his violence seemed exciting and gratifying for him. He smirked and openly laughed, relishing his audience, the control and my fear. The experience re-traumatised me and prevented me from moving on with my life. I think it cemented the impact of the original violence and now it shocks me to think that this happened.'

Abusive men do not make good role models. Yet there is still a widely held presumption in the family court – and in society as a whole – that contact with both parents is in the best interests of the child. Denying men any contact with children is incredibly rare – even if their abuse is clear. More often than not the courts do not consider the risk to the woman at all in relation to contact and residence. Lack of understanding about the impacts of domestic violence on children can lead some judges to award unsupervised contact to violent men. Welfare of children and their needs must be paramount in any decision – yet, in a recent Women's Aid survey, 44 per cent of women asked said that the family court granted contact to a former partner despite knowing that the child had been directly abused by them.[19] Tragically, some children pay the ultimate price for their father's need to control. Women's Aid's powerful report, *Nineteen Child Homicides*,[20] tells the stories of the children killed by domestic abuse perpetrators – their fathers – during formal or informal contact arrangements.

As of 2017, thankfully, changes to the family court are on the horizon. The Ministry of Justice has said family court judges will be given new powers to stop abusers from being able to torment their victims in court, and senior judges are taking steps to end the presumption that fathers must have contact with the child where there is evidence of domestic abuse that would put the child or mother at risk. There is even a change on the horizon that would give judges the power to appoint a legal aid solicitor to represent women without a lawyer; which – if enacted – would mean women like Diana are better supported.[21]

Once arrangements are agreed, these provide another opportunity for control. One study has found that more than half of women with post-separation contact arrangements with an abusive ex-partner continued to have serious, ongoing problems with this contact.[22] Take Felix and Andrea. Once she and Millie had moved out of the family home – and into a tiny flat – Felix was allowed to see his daughter at weekends. During 'his time', he would frequently take Millie away, including out of the country, without telling Andrea. 'I would have no idea where they were and be out of my mind with worry. He would never pick up the phone to let me know she was safe. He would take her to totally inappropriate places for a child, like gigs where he was getting drunk. It was like he saw her as his plaything.'

Andrea said, 'I remember once, over Easter, he just refused to bring Millie back. She was phoning me, telling me she wanted to come home early, but having monitored her mobile, he told me that he wasn't going to bring her back at all. It took days of negotiating before I eventually was allowed to drive for hours to collect her, at a time he designated – and of course he picked the day that was most inconvenient, when I was due to start a new job and Millie was about to start school. It's just so draining – it's constant mind games, and it costs money and time. It wears you down and it's unsettling for your child.'

# CHAPTER 3

# The Abused Woman

## What stops women leaving?

'Why does she stay with him?' is invariably the first question everyone asks when they hear that a woman is being abused by her partner. They think it should be so easy to walk out, slam the door and never return. But for most abused women it is not that simple.

Anyway, many women *do* leave. Refuge supports thousands of women every day who have done just that, but somehow we always find ourselves concentrating on the women who are unable to leave.

'Why does she stay?' is a question which always irritates me because I find it irrelevant. After all, if a woman's partner turns out to be a terrorist or an armed robber, would people immediately ask, 'Why does she stay with him?' In such a situation, people immediately recognise that such a man's behaviour cannot be tolerated, and should be prevented. So why should the focus be different when the issue is woman abuse?

Because the woman is the target of that abuse, you might say. But my whole thesis is that a woman does not cause her partner to be abusive any more than she might cause him to be a terrorist or a robber. And his behaviour – even if it does not involve physical abuse to the woman – should be just as intolerable to society.

Why a woman stays with an abusive man is not the point. The real issue is why do men abuse women in the first place and how can we prevent it from happening?

Whenever I hear someone say, 'Why does she stay?' I tell them they should turn the question around and ask, 'What stops her from leaving?' 'Why does she stay?' implies that there is something wrong with an abused woman, that she is somehow different from other women, that she is somehow responsible for ending the abuse. That of course is a myth: just as perfectly innocent airline passengers can become hostages in a hijack, a woman can unwittingly find herself in a relationship with an abusive man. And once she is caught up in the Charm Syndrome, it can be very hard indeed to get out. 'Why does she stay?' also suggests that a woman has complete control over her life – but it is Charm Syndrome Man, like a hijacker, who has all the real control.

It is important to understand the enormous odds a woman is up against, in order to see that the real point is not why she stays, but what a triumph it is when she is able to leave. Indeed, it is a miracle that she can cope with her predicament at all, at the same time as looking after her children, holding down a job, maintaining her sanity and so on. Imagine how you would feel if a violent attacker had the key to your front door, 365 days a year.

Never forget the power of the Charm Syndrome. One of the major effects of Charm Syndrome Man's behaviour is an overpowering sense of emotional dependency between him and his partner. He convinces her that the two of them are bound together in a kind of symbiotic relationship, in which each depends on the other for their very existence. This dependency is so powerful that most women don't want their relationships to end. It is only the bad times which they want stopped.

After a period of abuse, most women quite naturally are looking for respite, reassurance and calm. Because they are usually so isolated, they feel that there is often no one who can offer a shoulder – except their abusers themselves. As Melinda told me, whenever she needed comfort after the abuse, there was Trevor putting his arms around her, telling her he would look after her. When their partners reveal the comforting, tender and loving side of their characters in this way it is hardly surprising that the women are drawn back towards them.

Charm Syndrome Man does not see 'his woman' as an individual, but as an extension of himself, and frequently she comes to believe that too – for better or for worse. She believes that *he* needs *her,* that without her he won't be able to cope. Many men threaten to commit suicide if their partners leave them, and the women believe they are capable of carrying out their threats.

When a man is violent and then pleads and cries and promises to change, it is all too easy – given how exhausted and confused an abused woman is – to believe him. Beverley told me that Dave had her trapped emotionally for a long time. 'He told me, or made me feel, that he might commit suicide, that he didn't know what would happen, he didn't know how he would cope, and obviously because I cared for him I didn't want to do him that damage,' she says.

'The whole situation is so complicated and complex. I should have left Dave years ago, for his sake too. As it was, I mothered him for 12 years and he became more and more helpless, so at 40 he ended up with no job and no money, nothing. But it's very difficult to leave somebody who you know loves you very much and is dependent on you, no matter how bad it is at times. Whenever he pleaded with me to forgive him, it really got to me. I could see how much he was hurting, and I wanted to make it all right.'

## Grief and loss

Ending a relationship is a painful and complex process for anyone, regardless of the circumstances. There will be ambivalent feelings, attempted reconciliations, hopes that things will improve, feelings of guilt at leaving, anxieties at facing a new life. An abused woman must also contend with the trauma of abuse and violence, as must her children.

She experiences the grief of separation. However unhappy and unsafe her home is, it is still an enormous wrench for a woman to leave the place in which her children were raised – the place in which she may have many happy memories of her relationship and family life. Any change is unsettling, let alone ending a relationship that has controlled and consumed every aspect of a woman's life. It can feel like a bereavement. She may grieve for the man with whom she had fallen in love and for the relationship they 'could' have had. Remember, an abused woman may see flashes of the charmer she first met right up until the moment she leaves and beyond – and Charm Syndrome Man is expert in placing the blame on her. A woman may well question what she could have done to make it work, and wonder whether, if only she had tried harder, the 'old' him might have returned. But the truth is that nothing a woman can do will alter her partner's behaviour.

## Fear and trauma

At other times it is pure fear which prevents a woman from leaving her partner – fear that he will come after her or her children if she tries to get away. This fear is not unfounded: as previously mentioned, women are at the greatest risk of homicide at the point of separation or after leaving a violent partner.[23] Indeed, one London study found that 76 per cent of domestic homicides involved separation[24] – the abuser strikes just as he feels he may be losing control. One woman, who had a small child and was pregnant again, told me she was scared to tell anyone about the times her husband battered her, because she believed that the children would be taken away. Many women are also terrified by the thought of having to go to the police or to take legal action against their partners.

Another fear is that of being alone. Many people are worried about being alone, but when a woman is being abused by her partner, this fear is often heightened because abusive men dominate and control their partners so much that they have convinced them that they are unable to cope on their own. These men have been at the centre of all their emotions – good and bad – for so long, how will they fill that vacuum? However badly treated they may be, fear of loneliness can often outweigh fear of abuse, particularly in situations where the battering is either infrequent or emotional and verbal rather than physical.

Melinda explains, 'I think it was fear that made me stay for so long, fear of a whole lot of things: fear of him finding me if I left, fear of failure, failing to make the relationship work. And during the last year I felt frightened of being on my own, which I had never been before. I was really bothered about it. How would I cope with the children, the practicalities of it? I felt frightened of losing the continuity, the kind of intimacy you have when you are living with someone.' For many women, there is also the fear of poverty. Her abuser might be the main breadwinner; they might have joint financial assets that would be hard to unravel; she may not want to leave their joint family home.

Ironically, even though she lived with a man who could viciously beat her at any time, Melinda was still more frightened of being without his protection against strangers. 'I would feel frightened that somebody was going to break in, that somebody was going to attack me, because I was on my own,' she says with a wry smile.

Even when there is no physical abuse involved, an abuser controls and dominates his partner so effectively that he can often convince her she is to blame for the abuse. So she is trapped by feelings of guilt and shame. She feels she must have done something to deserve her ill-treatment, so instead of leaving she tries to change. Or she lives in hope of her partner's charming side reappearing permanently.

Often it appears easier to stay than to accept defeat and face the outside world. 'There's still such a stigma about divorce,' says Rebecca, 'especially among the circles we moved in. Single women always seemed to be an embarrassment. Nobody knew quite what to do with them. There was always so much emphasis on couples that I felt that they would think I had failed if I left.' Society's disapproval of divorce and separation may have lessened since I first supported Rebecca, but so many women still tell me how they feel excluded from social events centred around couples. Not only do women lose a partner – who, for all the abuse, has been their 'other half' for many years – they often lose a circle of friends, and even in-laws to whom they may have been close.

If the woman has children, the issue is complicated still further because she may have been brought up to believe in the two-parent ideal at all costs. And Charm Syndrome Man exploits this to the full. Rebecca says, 'Ralph said to me that if we split up, my children would be deprived of a father again. He convinced me that it would have a detrimental effect on them.'

An abused woman may be frightened of independence, of being without a man. Women constantly say to me: 'How will I survive without him?' 'Will I ever find anybody else?' 'I'm 40 and not used to being single.' They say these things because they have been brought up to think in this way. They may even stay to preserve their husband's reputation, to avoid ruining his career.

Abused women are frequently isolated from friends and family. They have no one to turn to and nowhere to go. They may have little or no contact with an outside world which could show them their predicament from a different viewpoint. Even career women who have contact with people every day still feel so humiliated and ashamed by the fact that the person they are closest to is treating them abusively that they keep their problems to themselves. The result is that they are more dependent than ever on their abusers.

They do not stay with their partners because they are some kind of masochist, or because they just give up and give in. They are often very angry, but their partners have prevented them from expressing their anger for so long that they are unable to use it constructively: to hold him responsible for his abuse, for example, or take steps towards leaving the relationship.

Melinda, like many women in her position, see-sawed between wanting to reach out to Trevor to comfort and be comforted, and feeling so angry and frustrated that she fantasised about revenge. 'I would plot these kinds of fantasy ways I could make him suffer, or ways I could eradicate him or blot him out by killing him,' she admits. 'I would lie awake at night and watch him sleeping and I would imagine shooting him or plunging a knife into him, and I was quite obsessed by the feeling. Or I would fantasise that he'd been in an accident on the motorway and killed or disabled, because if it happened like that I would not get found out, whereas if I attacked him in some way, I'd be guilty.'

Many women feel this way. They feel they have so little control over their situation, that the only way out is to actually kill their partners or themselves, or somehow to will their abusers to go off with another woman or walk under a bus. Odd as it may sound, when women are in this state of desperation and confusion, of suppressed anger and fear, leaving does not seem final enough. They feel that just walking out of the door will not end the nightmare. Their partners will still come after them and threaten them, or persuade them to come home. As Melinda says, 'I felt as if Trevor had some kind of spell over me. That the only way I would ever be free of him was if he was dead.'

## Stress and anxiety

No matter how often abused women dream of revenge, they rarely inflict any physical violence on their partners, however angry and bitter they may feel. Instead they tend to internalise the anger, often becoming so stressed and worn out that it is all they can do to cope from day to day, without also having to consider the enormous strain of actually trying to leave their partners. Such women have been so controlled and dominated that they have grown used to suppressing their feelings, and they often lack the self-confidence to make any decisions at all. They are frequently debilitated by a catalogue of illnesses and complaints, especially the kind of psychosomatic ailments associated with stress, such as backache, headache and fatigue. 'Over a period of time,' says Beverley, 'it was as if my body knew things were not right, things were not as they should be, and it was giving me very strong messages. For a period of about one or two years, on long weekends, or if we spent three or four days together, I would have low back pain and I would be constipated and this became a really well-established pattern.'

They may suffer from insomnia, agoraphobia or anxiety, or find themselves constantly on edge. When a woman spends every moment anticipating the next blow or barrage of abuse from her abuser – and how she might avoid it – imagine the distress she endures. Imagine how it feels to be seriously assaulted once a week for six years. What would be left of your sense of self, your sense of purpose, your hopes for the future?

Since I first wrote this book, there is more understanding and recognition of the psychological impact that domestic violence has on a woman. The World Health Organization has found that women who experience domestic violence are twice as likely to experience depression.[25] In Refuge's own services, 22 per cent of women who responded to a mental health screening measure had made plans to end their own lives. Almost half say they feel depressed. Fourteen per cent arrive with issues around drug misuse. And these are the women who *have* managed to seek support. When a woman is this traumatised, worn out or depressed, is it any wonder that frequently she does not have the emotional energy to put together a plan of escape?

The grinding, psychological impact of abuse must not be underestimated. All too often, women experiencing domestic violence end up taking their own lives – every week, an estimated three women die in this way.[26] Isolated from social supports, they lose hope of any sense of a 'future'. They feel trapped and defeated, unable to envisage a life free from abuse. Suicide can seem like the only way out of a situation in which a woman believes there is no hope of change and no possibility of escape.

Take the case of Gurda Dhaliwal, who experienced decades of abuse from her husband. Her brother, Nav Jagpal, told me: 'The first few years seemed fine, but as it went on, his abuse became more apparent. He would have a go at her the moment people left, or just before people arrived. He controlled the way she had to act in front of others. Even at that point, as an 11-year-old boy, I could tell the difference in her behaviour when he was in the room or even in the house, compared to when he wasn't. When she was free of him, she could relax and speak openly.' Gurda's story is heartbreakingly familiar – you can see it echoed in the cases throughout this book – yet, tragically, Gurda never got the protection she needed. On 22 February 2005, she walked to the outbuilding at the bottom of her garden and hanged herself. When her body was found, she had a gash across her forehead and bruises on her arms.

When a woman feels there is no way out, and the pain of abuse becomes too unbearable, it is easy to see why she might perceive that the only option is the destruction of herself.

However, for a small minority of women living with life-threatening physical and sexual abuse, the destruction of the *perpetrator* represents a final chance of escape. I have acted as an expert witness in murder and manslaughter cases when the accused is an abused woman. My role has been to ensure the jury understands the woman's state of mind at the time of the offence. Johnson and Ferraro describe how most abused women 'experience a turning point when the violence or abuse done to them comes to be felt as a basic threat, whether to their physical, or social self, or both'.[27] The turning point may come when the woman notices an escalation in the severity of abuse and recognises that she is in great danger. In his book, Professor Charles Ewing describes how a woman who lives in a state of pervasive fear, which consumes all of her thoughts and energy, may come to see that if she doesn't assert herself, she may risk losing herself.[28] In some women's perception, killing her abuser is the only way to avoid the destruction of her psychological self.

For many women, leaving is not an option. These women may one day face a stark choice: to be killed or to kill. They are driven by intolerable circumstances to act drastically to end their victimisation. Sandra Fleming is one such woman. Sandra suffered torture, physical violence and degradation at the hands of her husband, Christopher Porter. One night in 1993, Christopher threatened Sandra with his loaded Luger pistol. He also pointed the gun at their eldest daughter, threatening to shoot her if Fleming left. In a state of absolute terror, Sandra shot and killed him. She pleaded guilty to manslaughter on the grounds of diminished responsibility – an 'abnormality of mind' – and was placed on probation for three years. Sandra was a normal person, yet nothing could have been more abnormal than the situation in which she found herself.

When it comes to the mental health of women who have suffered abuse, I want to make one thing absolutely clear: even though a woman may be suffering depression or suicidal thoughts, it is important not to blur the distinction between being mentally ill and being traumatised as a result of violence. When abused women are labelled as mad, they are 'othered' – the myth that domestic violence only happens to certain types of 'vulnerable' women is perpetuated, and the perpetrator's responsibility is reduced. As Mary Ann Dutton writes in her book on the physical and psychological impacts of abuse, 'the battered women are not "sick", but they are in a "sick" situation.'[29] Women are simply reacting in a normal way to abnormal and dangerous circumstances.

## Where would they go?

Aside from the trauma and day-to-day stress of coping with abuse, there are practical barriers that stop women leaving. Many women are dependent on their abusers not only emotionally but also financially since the men insist on handling – or, as is often the case, mishandling – the financial aspect of a relationship. The abused woman may be tied to the home with young children, or her partner may have refused to allow her to take a job and earn an independent wage. The result is that the woman often has no funds of her own to enable her to leave. Many women tell me their husbands have threatened to sell the house if they leave, so they will not even have a roof over their heads.

Rebecca says, 'Ralph dug his heels in and insisted he would never leave *his* home, so what could I do? I couldn't physically throw him out. When I threatened to get a solicitor, Ralph just laughed in my face. After all, he is one himself – and he knew all the tricks. He would have had an answer for everything. As always!'

When I talk to abused women at Refuge, I am constantly aware of their appalling plight with regard to housing. There is a national housing shortage. A woman who wants to leave her abusive partner must contend with high rents and short tenancies in the private rental sector when she may already be locked into paying a mortgage or rent on her current property. Add to the mix the fact that she is likely to have faced some form of financial abuse. How is she meant to scrape together enough for a deposit on a new property so she can break away? The waiting lists for council housing have never been longer. An abused woman – even with support from a charity like Refuge – may struggle to demonstrate that she and her children are eligible for a new, safe home; or she may be moved to an entirely different part of the country. Is it any wonder that researchers have found that 70 per cent of female rough sleepers have experienced domestic violence?[30]

A woman's only alternative may be to seek help from a refuge – if she even knows that they exist. Yet England and Wales have never had enough refuge provision. The Council of Europe recommends that there is one family place in a refuge per 10,000 of the population.[31] We have always fallen well below this. At the time of writing, Refuge runs more than 40 safe houses, but we regularly have to deal with cuts from our funders – often local authorities dealing with their own much-reduced budgets – and we fundraise tirelessly in order to keep the doors open. Women's Aid – which acts as a federation body for many UK refuges – estimated that England lost 25 per cent of its specialist service provision between 2010 and 2014.[32] In some parts of the country there is now no refuge provision at all. Refuge recently stepped in to save a local refuge when it faced closure – but we do not have the resources to do this everywhere. Many women and children, often fleeing in fear for their lives, are turned away from refuges on a daily basis, simply because there is not the bed space. Many abused women and children have no escape route. They are faced with an impossible choice: they can flee to the streets with their children, or remain with their abuser and risk further violence – or worse.

One woman I met had been driving around in a van for months with her little daughter because there was literally nowhere for her to go. Another woman, whose husband was a dentist, was forced to leave him and take her four children to the local housing department after he had been so violent that she feared for all their lives. She was told there was absolutely nothing available: not bed and breakfast, not even a bed space in a homeless families' hostel. The result was that her four children were taken from her and put into care while she was left to fend for herself. She was so desperate that the only thing she could think of was to take the train to Gatwick, where there were cafés open and where she could curl up and sleep unnoticed. Another woman had been trying to get a bed space in a refuge for three weeks – she had been calling everywhere but was too frightened to contact the police or social services for fear her four children would be taken away. Instead, she slept on a park bench in the pouring rain with her children.

Again and again, I support women with no money, nowhere to go, no one to turn to. Is it any wonder many women are faced with little option but to return home to their abusers? Women should never be judged for making that impossible decision. Even if a refuge space *is* available, the barriers do not end there. Some women are unaware of the state benefits they can claim or they are reluctant to put themselves in a position of being dependent on 'handouts'. Research by Refuge found that half of women accessing its services had experienced financial abuse and the majority of those women were what the government considers to be 'financially excluded'. Around one-third do not have a bank account. Often, when they arrive at our doors, women have little more than the clothes on their backs.

When a woman is ready to leave a refuge, it may be that the only housing available is in a completely new area, away from new friends she and her children have made. The children frequently feel unsettled because invariably they have to change schools. Often they are put into temporary accommodation and then moved on, causing even more disruption in their lives. Sometimes the children become so desperate for home comforts, their own friends and their toys that the women give in and go home to their partners rather than upset the children any more.

Then there is the question of how they will make ends meet. Women who have stayed at home for years with young children may worry about who will care for them if they have to go out to work: they may not have friends or family who can help; childcare facilities in some areas are woefully scarce; and private nurseries are very expensive.

## Locked out of support

Some women are not entitled to any support whatsoever – they have 'no recourse to public funds'. They may be in the UK on spousal visas, with their immigration status reliant on their abusive husband. They may have been trafficked and forced into marriage or prostitution, or they may have overstayed student or work visas. All abused women feel trapped, but for these women the options for escape are vanishingly small. They may have no claim to social housing or benefits; or documents to enable them to work; and their perpetrators will often use the threat of reporting them to the authorities as a means of further control and abuse.

Anh got in touch with Refuge through its specialist service for Vietnamese women. Ten years before she came to Refuge, Anh had been trafficked into forced labour and was petrified by her abusers' threats of deportation if she tried to escape. The traffickers regularly subjected her to physical, financial and psychological abuse and said that her immigration status meant nobody would help her. Once she had been brought to safety, Anh told Refuge she found it difficult to look in the mirror because all she could see was the reflection of a very old and grey person. She worried constantly about her health deteriorating and feared that nobody would be able to identify her if she died or had an accident. Her identity had been so eroded by her abusers that she feared nobody would know who she was.

When women like this are referred to Refuge, we do everything in our power to make them safe. Our expert staff will support them to make asylum applications so that they can begin to claim benefits and we will find them a safe place to stay. But we cannot reach everyone. Many women will end up sleeping on the sofas of friends or acquaintances, or on the streets. Some abused women who are in the UK on spousal visas may now apply for leave to remain in the country, independent of their perpetrator – but this will only be granted if they can prove that their partners abused them. 'Evidence' of abuse might mean a letter from a GP, or a police report – documents any woman struggles to get her hands on, let alone a woman who does not speak English, or who has never before come into contact with statutory agencies in this country.

One Latin American woman, whose husband beat her up after only a couple of months of marriage, came to Refuge for help. Even though she was pregnant, because of her foreign status she was incorrectly told she was not entitled to state benefits or housing. To cap it all, she was advised that if after a year she was no longer living with her husband, the Home Office would have her deported. Her only options were either to become dependent yet again, this time on Refuge, or return to her husband and not only face more abuse but be labelled by society as a masochist for 'going back for more'.

Even if they are entitled to benefits, women from ethnic minority backgrounds often face immense difficulties in accessing support. In the Asian community, separation and divorce are still so frowned upon that a woman may fear being ostracised for contacting the police or leaving her husband. As a result, she may feel particularly isolated and alone. An Asian woman I supported had four children, all of them girls. Each time she gave birth to a girl, her husband beat her for not producing a boy. After the birth of her fourth daughter, there was a particularly violent assault. One day, he deliberately started a fire in the kitchen. Her nine-year-old ran out of the house to a neighbour across the street to get help, but by the time she got back, the house was in flames. Unbeknown to the young girl, her mother had managed to get her children into the garden before the flames took hold. You would think these would be more than reasonable grounds for divorce, wouldn't you? However, her family told her it was not permitted. She was forced to return to her husband but was told that if he beat her again, she could leave. Sure enough, his abuse continued as soon as she returned. A couple of months later, she began divorce proceedings. Following the divorce, she was shunned by her community. Nobody would speak to her; she was refused service in the local shop and verbally abused in the street.

If a woman from an ethnic minority background does obtain protection from agencies, she may find herself facing language barriers and ingrained prejudices. The case of Sabina Akhtar – a Bangladeshi woman who arrived in the UK to live with her husband, Malik Mannan, a British national who murdered Sabina in 2008 – shows how dangerous this can be. Weeks before her death, Sabina had gone to the police to report her husband's assaults and threats that he would kill her. No formal statement was taken or complaint lodged owing to her perceived confusion and language difficulties. The next day, following another attack, Malik *was* arrested before being released on police bail on condition that he stay away from Sabina. He did not, and continued to contact and harass her. During this period, Sabina was wrongly informed that she would not be able to get divorced in the UK because she had got married in Bangladesh. When Malik turned up at her home, banging on the front door and shouting through the letterbox, he was arrested again for breaching bail conditions. Yet the Crown Prosecution Service decided not to charge. He was released with all bail conditions dropped. Five days later he stabbed Sabina to death in her home in front of their two-year-old son.

Malik was convicted of Sabina's murder and was sentenced to life imprisonment with an order to serve a minimum of 17 years. The jury found him guilty in 20 minutes – the quickest verdict in the history of Manchester Crown Court at the time. Later, at the inquest, the coroner concluded that 'serious and significant failings' had been made by Greater Manchester Police, Manchester Social Services and the Crown Prosecution Service, which 'possibly' contributed to Sabina's death. Sabina's son is now safe. Sabina's heartbroken uncle, Reaz Talukder, told me: 'Sabina was loved very dearly by her family and friends – she was a brave woman and devoted to her son. We are determined to fight against the injustice that other women like Sabina experience.' Clearly, Sabina was a high-risk victim. Many women have fallen victim to similar injustices, and vulnerable children have lost their mothers in such circumstances, but I have shared Sabina's story because it clearly demonstrates how women from minority ethnic backgrounds may have an even higher mountain to climb when it comes to agencies taking them seriously.

If these women do successfully access support, what happens afterwards? One black woman told me she feels doubly abused: by her partner and by a society which can still be prejudiced, particularly when it comes to employment. Consider that in 2015, the gender pay gap was 19.2 per cent, and the ethnicity pay gap was 5 per cent; and that across Great Britain, race remains the most commonly recorded motivation for hate crime.[33]

Another woman, who desperately wanted to do a further education course at college to enable her to get a good job, found herself blocked at every turn. Because she was staying at Refuge she had moved boroughs. Her former borough accepted her for the course, but the fees were unaffordable because she was no longer a local resident. She begged and borrowed the money to pay the fees and arranged for a friend to look after her child. Unfortunately, those plans fell through. She applied to the local authority in the new borough for childcare, and was told there were no facilities; and even if there had been, she would not have been eligible because she was not a permanent resident. She could not afford private childcare, so in the end she was forced to give up the course. The only saving grace was that we were able to find her housing, though she still has to live on state benefits, much against her principles.

Even when a woman is determined to leave, if she cannot afford solicitors' fees she may find it extremely hard to get legal aid because there are such strict rules about eligibility. Women have to prove that they are on a low income, which involves time and a lot of red tape at a period of their lives when such obstacles are especially demoralising. The legal aid budget has been drastically reduced since 2004, so the eligibility criteria have become much stricter. Women must also produce evidence that the domestic abuse occurred, and that it happened within a certain time frame. Of the women who enter Refuge's services in need of legal aid, only a small fraction succeed in getting it. How is an abused woman – already worn out and disheartened – supposed to access justice without any support? The result is that some abused women are forced to represent themselves in child-related proceedings; and, as previously mentioned, they may face their abusers in court and may even be questioned by them. One woman I supported was cross-examined by her QC husband. Where is the justice in that? Alternatively, women are forced to sell their homes in order to pay for legal representation. Another scenario is that they feel pressured into attending mediation sessions where they must sit across the table from the abuser, who has systematically dominated them, in order to 'work things out'. I am seriously concerned about the current move towards restorative justice programmes for all victims of crime. Of course, 'restorative' contact with the perpetrator of a crime may be beneficial for some victims – for a person burgled by a stranger, hearing their remorse may reduce their fear, for example – but it can never be appropriate in cases of domestic or sexual violence. The abuser's methods of control can be so subtle, so insidious, that any 'restorative' meeting may offer another opportunity for abuse or re-traumatise the woman.

It is easy to say glibly, 'Women have a choice – why don't they leave if it's so bad?' But do they really have a choice? Sometimes I wonder how the abused women who come to our refuges have managed to leave at all, given the emotional, financial, psychological and social obstacles they have to overcome. Abused women are trapped. They are women who are frightened, confused, isolated. Yet they are survivors; resilient, courageous women who in the face of a living hell cope admirably. In fact it is often because they are so preoccupied with coping and surviving in the short term that they are unable to distance themselves long enough to make the long-term decision to leave.

## Survivors, not victims

'You can't win, so you soon learn that it's easier just to shut up than find yourself being hit or abused again,' says Hazel. An abused woman is in a situation remarkably similar to that described by hostages: her life may be in the balance; she is isolated from outside help; and the person who is in control of her life can switch to being charming, kind and comforting.

This is a very similar scenario to the one in which four employees of a Stockholm bank found themselves in August 1973, after robbers burst in and held them as hostages. Unexpectedly, these hostages feared the police more than their captors. They even developed a kind of bond with the robbers. Sociologists studying this incident called it the Stockholm Syndrome: when the hostages survived, they felt that they were indebted to their captors for giving them back their lives. According to these sociologists there is a parallel between the relationship of hostage and captor, and the kind of dependency which often occurs between a battered woman and her abuser.

Certainly, like the hostages, abused women often find themselves in ambivalent situations, not knowing whether to hate their partners or to try to reach out to them, but instinctively justifying and defending them in preference to trusting outsiders. I would say that both the Stockholm hostages and abused women behave this way because they are acting out of natural instincts for self-preservation. Consciously or subconsciously, they are aiming to survive.

It is easy to be sceptical when you are not trapped in such a position – but think about it. When a woman has been relentlessly criticised, made to feel worthless and cut off from her friends and outside support, is it any wonder that she is unable to challenge her abuser, any more than a hostage is likely to defy a captor who has a gun pointed at his or her head?

By appearing submissive and going along with their captors' wishes, abused women – like the hostages – realise, often instinctively, that they can buy themselves time while they think of a long-term strategy or an escape plan.

'Compliance' can be a way of surviving, a way of getting through their ordeal physically and emotionally intact.

Many sociologists disagree. They believe that abused women are in a state of 'learned helplessness', a syndrome described by Lenore Walker in *The Battered Woman*.[34] Walker suggests that battered women believe that they cannot control their situation, so they become passive, submissive and helpless. The theory is based on experiments performed on various animals, particularly those carried out by experimental psychologist Martin Seligman on dogs.

The dogs were put into cages and given electric shocks at random intervals. At first the dogs reacted, but when they realised that nothing they did prevented the shocks they became passive and gave up trying. Even when the cage doors were opened, the dogs still did not respond. Finally, they had to be repeatedly dragged to their escape routes before they began to react for themselves again. The longer the dogs had been exposed to the shocks, the longer it took them to recover from the effects of this 'learned helplessness'. According to those who subscribe to the theory, abused women behave in much the same way.

In my experience, however, though women may be temporarily paralysed by abuse, often finding it difficult to make decisions or solve problems, very few give up trying to change their situation. Unlike Seligman's dogs, they do not easily accept defeat. To the outside world, because they do not immediately dash for the door, they may seem submissive and passive, but in fact, in all sorts of often subtle ways, they fight back, they adopt survival techniques and actively find ways of coping.

Imagine for a moment a scene from one of those old-fashioned cinema melodramas. The heroine is on a train, being driven by her handsome husband, who, she has discovered too late, is a murderer. She knows that after 100 miles the train is going to smash into the buffers and both of them will die, but 100 miles seems a long way off, and she knows she must survive until then. The immediate way of achieving this seems to be to find a good hiding place, so that he can't find her and attack her, while she thinks of what to do next. People along the railway line are shouting: 'Why doesn't she jump off? She must like the danger,' they reckon, 'otherwise she'd escape.' And by now the woman is so frightened that she too wishes she had jumped off at the beginning, but the train seems to be hurtling along faster than ever, and it is far too difficult…or is it? Maybe it isn't too late to jump after all…

Just as she is considering jumping, her husband finds her. But instead of attacking her, as she expects, he says: 'Stay with me, I need you. If you stay, I'll steer the train to HAPPY EVER AFTER.' The woman is by now terrified and confused, but she is still able to grasp at straws. HAPPY EVER AFTER is where she always wanted to live, after all. The relief of not having to jump off the dangerously speeding train, and the fact that her husband now seems remorseful, gentle and kind, and is offering her warmth and love makes this seem the better option.

But, just as she is beginning to relax, she realises that the change of direction was only a loop line, and that she is back on the main line to CHAOS, with her husband laughing and threatening her once more, and the train travelling faster than ever...She realises she has no choice: she has to jump and risk the consequences. When she recovers from her leap, she is confused and bruised, but she is safe and FREE.

A pretty dramatic analogy, certainly, yet when a woman lives with an abuser she behaves in a similar fashion. All her energies are devoted to immediate, short-term survival. It is difficult for her to see the picture as a whole: the idea of leaving her partner is as nerve-racking and dangerous as jumping from that train. Yet, like the woman on the train, rather than being a pathetic, passive victim, she is a resourceful and coping survivor.

The abused woman is in a situation over which she has little control, yet she cannot accept that; she believes she can change things, that by altering her own behaviour she can bring out the loving side of her partner, the side she fell in love with. So she adopts every strategy she can think up. It is only when she finally realises that she cannot alter her abuser's behaviour, that – however charming and gentle he is capable of being at times – he will always revert to abusive behaviour, only then can she summon up the strength and courage to jump off the train.

It is a mistake to assume that abused women do not fight back or stand up for themselves. The women I talk to adopt all kinds of strategies to survive. Sometimes they are subconscious, almost reflex actions, sometimes they are deliberate plans for survival.

The most universal instinctive way that women cope at one time or another during their relationship is to do what their husbands and boyfriends do: they minimise the problem, deny it altogether or actually forget that it happened – because it is simply too painful or problematical to deal with. This is known as denial and I will go into it in more detail in the next chapter.

Hazel, like many abused women, had her own special survival tactics. She had hair long enough to sit on, but after her husband grabbed it and pulled her around the house by it on several occasions she had it cut short to prevent him from doing it again. Another ploy was always to sit on the chair nearest the door – 'ready to run'.

Laura hid the kitchen knives, while Beverley kept a set of clothes in a bag near the stairs and another in the battered car she refused to sell – just in case. 'I was holding on to my sanity,' she says, 'I was holding on to my possessions, which I thought were my life.'

One woman told me that when her husband started a row the first thing he would do was reach for the wooden hangers in the wardrobe and hit her with one – so she replaced them all with plastic ones. Another woman was repeatedly raped by her husband, who came home every night drunk. One night she hid a carving knife under her pillow and, after he raped her, she held it to his throat and said, 'If you ever do that again, I'll kill you.' After that, she moved into the spare room and they never slept together again. This woman came off lightly – most abusers take revenge if their partners challenge them in this way.

Abused women often cope by adopting their partner's political and social views, to steer clear of confrontation, or they adapt their behaviour, avoiding scenarios which have led to verbal or physical assaults in the past. Like the hostages in the Stockholm bank, they appear to outsiders to be colluding with their abusers, yet they are acting almost instinctively out of a sense of self-preservation.

Hazel says, 'I used to keep my face timid and say nothing, so he couldn't put me in the wrong and have an excuse for hitting me. You learn over the years not to challenge them, so they don't kick you about. Sometimes I'd curl up in a ball, hide in a corner, just to try and stay out of his way. I was forever saying to my family, "Don't say that because he'll get annoyed and don't do this because he won't like it..."'

One woman adopted a whole set of survival tactics, ranging from carrying a key to her neighbour's house in her pocket at all times, to deliberately keeping quiet, never speaking unless her husband spoke first, so that he could not accuse her of starting an argument. 'I got clever, I had been with him so long,' she says. 'When he started shouting and hitting me, I'd stay as long as I could to make sure the kids were all right, and to see if he'd calm down. If he didn't, I'd put my coat on and say I had to go out for cigarettes. I had arranged a secret meeting place with the kids – at a café nearby – so whenever I had to leave, they knew where to find me. I also made an arrangement with my next-door neighbour that if ever she heard screams, she would call the police.'

Many women learn to lie, to be deceitful, to avoid their partner's displeasure. Jimmy would be furious if Hazel wasted food. 'He got cross if something went bad in the fridge and I hadn't used it,' she says. 'He'd shout, "It's a waste, it's a waste!", so if I did find something, I'd wrap it up in tin-foil and hide it in the bottom of the bin with something over the top of it. You become very secretive – not because you're a secretive person but to avoid their wrath.'

If Rebecca was busy with the children and unable to have the supper ready by the time Ralph came home, she would put a stockpot onto the stove so that the smell would fool him into thinking his meal was cooking. 'Otherwise,' she said, 'there would be a row.'

The point about survival techniques is that they are never long-term solutions. They help the woman cope with her immediate predicament while she gathers the strength and makes plans for the final separation. But they can never solve the problem, because *nothing* a woman does can alter an abuser's behaviour. Only *he* can do that.

Sally, Melinda, Rebecca, Hazel, Beverley and Laura, like all abused women, had to make up their minds to leave in their own time. First they had to recognise that coping and surviving is only a short-term measure – that, by being brave, abused women simply become part of the denial conspiracy.

# Chapter 4

# The Denial Conspiracy

## Whose problem is it anyway?

One of the most striking aspects of the problem of woman abuse is that there seems to be a great conspiracy on the part of the men involved, and on the part of society as a whole, to pretend that woman abuse is not really a problem at all.

### *'He denied everything'*

Abusive men frequently deny their abuse outright, suggesting that the women are making it up or that they are crazy. To the police, neighbours, family, they will say, 'Of course it isn't true. She's imagining it.' And, because they can be so charming, they sound only too plausible. Hazel says, 'Jimmy denied everything. If Jimmy said something didn't happen, it didn't happen. I mean, he denied ever hitting me, and as far as he's concerned, he hasn't.'

Guy, like many abusers, simply lied whenever Sally suspected he was having an affair (which he was), making her feel guilty for even suggesting such a thing. 'One day,' she remembers, 'a woman phoned up and seemed confused when I answered the phone. It seemed she was the mother of one of his mistresses – she claimed that Guy was actually engaged to her daughter! I can still hear her now saying, "That man is like a ram rushing up and down the countryside!"

'When Guy came home I confronted him with what she had said, but he told me this girl was some crazy student who had a crush on him. He told me that in his position these things happened all the time, and I shouldn't give it a second thought. It was me he loved, etcetera, etcetera. And, probably because I wanted to, I believed it. Do you know, I found out later that he had actually been dating hundreds of women!'

Melinda says, 'Trevor would absolutely dispute that he was ever physically violent – even though he had knocked me down, kicked and slapped me. He said it was just my fears and fantasies. I even had a friend who had been physically abused by her husband – much worse than me. She had had broken arms and broken legs, and Trevor was very sympathetic towards her. I tried to say that she wasn't very different to me – even though I had no broken bones, the way he made me feel was the same: the fear, the intimidation and the frustration. But he couldn't see it.'

Even if Charm Syndrome Man does not actually deny his actions outright or insist that his partner is crazy, he will deny responsibility by minimising the seriousness of his behaviour, and suggesting that his partner is overreacting or exaggerating. 'I barely touched her – she just bruises easily', 'It was only a little slap', or 'I didn't hit her *that* hard' are well-used lines.

Even if an abuser admits to his behaviour, he will make excuses. 'It wasn't my fault – I was drunk' or 'You know I didn't mean it – I'd just had a bad day at work and I took it out on her' are typical. Charm Syndrome Man will blame alcohol, a sudden loss of temper, jealousy, the fact that he is unemployed, miserable at work or worried about money – anything and everyone but himself. And, more often than not, first in line for the blame is the woman he has abused.

Even if a man accepts what he has done, he will often attempt to *justify* it. 'I was provoked,' he will say, or 'She brings out the worst in me.'

## *'I told myself it wasn't really that bad'*

It is not only the man who denies and minimises his behaviour – the woman frequently does the same thing, partly from fear of recrimination from her partner – remember how Trevor threatened to kill Melinda if she ever told anyone – and partly because they are afraid of facing up to the problem because, once they do so, they will have to face up to difficult and painful feelings.

They will have to admit that the person they love – or once loved – most, the charmer who seemed so wonderful, is somebody entirely different: callous, unreliable, controlling. And once they recognise that, they feel they must do something about it. How can they accept all this and not act? They are caught in a double bind: to leave or to stay, when neither option seems to be the answer. Rather than face such decisions, it seems easier to justify, excuse and minimise their partners' behaviour. The irony is that by doing so they allow their abusers to get away with it.

Many women (as I suggested in the previous chapter) use denial as a positive way of surviving from day to day, while they gather strength to leave. It is a tactic often adopted by people in difficult and distasteful jobs. They push away painful feelings. If they crack up, they feel, they will be no use to anyone, so they temporarily shut out the greater implications and dangers of their situation and concentrate on the particular job in hand.

One psychologist calls this 'psychic numbing'[35] and likens it to the behaviour of the survivors of Hiroshima, who, though they were perfectly aware of the devastation all around them, found a way of coping by closing themselves off and numbing themselves to the horror.

When Guy denied that he had been unfaithful to Sally, she says, 'Subconsciously, I trained myself to believe it. You've got to survive and avoid aggravation. And if he had admitted that he had had affairs, I felt I would have fallen apart. I couldn't stay with someone who was unfaithful. I would have had to do something about it, and I suppose I wasn't ready to face up to that.

'I even managed to let him convince me of the most bizarre things! On one occasion I came home from work to find a used condom in the waste-paper bin in the bedroom. He came in at that moment and when he realised I had seen it he actually said he'd been masturbating and didn't want to stain the sheets! When I look back, it's incredible that I preferred to let myself go along with it, rather than cause another row. It is amazing the way he managed to put his own slant on everything.'

When women first come to me for support, it can take a long time before they are actually able to remember many of the things that have disturbed them most. For many women 'forgetting' these things is a way of coping, while they gather the strength to deal with their predicament. Even after they have been talking to me for a period of time, there is still this inclination to 'forget' the bad times. There would be occasions when I would have to remind Melinda that Trevor had beaten and abused her, because in the interim periods he had been so caring and attentive that, consciously or unconsciously, she had blocked out the bad memories.

'It frightens me now,' she agrees, 'but during the good times I lost my ability to remember the abuse. I would try and think about the times when he had hit and kicked me, and in a way I would find myself believing Trevor's perception of it. It was as if I had imagined it, that it didn't really happen or that it couldn't have been that bad.

'Even the extreme situations like the time after my mum's funeral when he threatened to push me under the train, and the time when I had a miscarriage and he shouted at me and told me he was going to leave me, and he was aggressive and abusive for three weeks afterwards. Those kinds of things I just couldn't remember, until after the relationship ended, and then they all kept flooding back. I would be doing something and suddenly I'd remember and think, "Oh God, what about the time he did that..."

'I had always thought that I could speak up for myself against any wrongs or injustices that were being done to me, but in this kind of crazy situation I didn't. Because I felt so incredibly reduced as a person, and because I found it so hard to accept that I was in this situation, I suppose I went along with Trevor's view of things, because it was a way of coping. If I was going to stay with him, then I *had* to believe it. I was so completely confused about who I was and what my feelings were that it seemed easier in a way to cope with the outside world by isolating myself and not expressing what was happening.'

Often women keep quiet about abuse, because their partner's controlling behaviour has ensured that they feel too guilty and ashamed to admit what is happening. Rebecca says, 'I didn't tell anyone for a long time, because I was embarrassed. I didn't want anyone to know that this so-called perfect relationship was really nothing of the kind.'

'The shame was very, very strong,' says Laura. 'I was terribly middle-class. To my friends I developed this strategy of not talking about things. I just told them the same old story about everything being fine. I was reluctant to tell anyone because I wanted people to see us as a pair and a family. I didn't want to admit what was really happening. Also, I had the whole thing about feeling guilt – you know, thinking I must have brought it on myself somehow.'

Melinda says, 'I was so ashamed of it that I didn't tell anybody until the last time when Trevor marked my face so badly that I couldn't hide it. You tend to block out the bad things. You can't actually remember the details. And I think I had the idea that no marriage is totally wonderful all the time. That's what I told myself.'

Most relationships, of course, *aren't* wonderful all the time – but there is a difference between a healthy relationship which has its ups and downs and one where a man consistently abuses his partner, where he makes her afraid to be herself and unable to do the things she wants to do, and where she has to deny and minimise whole chunks of her life.

Blaming herself is another way of minimising and denying in order to cope. If a woman feels she is to blame for her partner's behaviour, it follows that by altering her behaviour she can stop the abuse. In believing this, a woman can believe that she still has some element of control over her situation. For many women, the idea of accepting that they are completely powerless to change their partners' behaviour is just too frightening to accept.

### 'He must have had a good reason'

So the abusers and the abused deny – but society also denies and minimises the problem of woman abuse by going along with Charm Syndrome Man's excuses. It is easier for society to believe that a man abuses a woman because he has had too much to drink or is jealous than to take a long hard look at itself and see whether, perhaps, there is more to it than that. If it did see that, it would have to do something about it. Often, too, like the survivors of Hiroshima, society finds it easier to pretend that the abuse is not happening, to 'numb' itself to the reality, because it is simply too appalling to face.

Society also denies the problem in its reluctance to become involved in what happens between a man and a woman behind closed doors. People feel awkward and embarrassed, and do not want to interfere. 'A man's home is his castle,' we say, as usual, and regard interference as an invasion of privacy.

Friends and families are often reluctant to intervene in cases of physical abuse – even though these same people would probably rush to dial 999 if they saw a stranger being attacked on the street. And as long as the community turns a blind eye in this way, a man's castle will often be a woman's prison. I find this attitude extraordinary. After all, if a burglar were to say, 'Sorry, I only rob people when I've had a bad day at work or I'm on drugs', who would listen?

There are some people, of course, who think women are not really that important anyway. In the debate over whether or not to abolish mandatory life sentences for murder, a *Times* editorial (25 September 1989) noted that 'murderers vary from remorseful men who, when quarrelling with their wives, have gripped or hit too hard – to robbers going armed with intent to shoot their way to their spoils if necessary'. In other words, there are murders and there are murders, and when a man murders his partner it is a 'crime of passion' which is somehow excusable.

Of course, these days, some men are careful not to flaunt their sexism so readily. In fact, many a modern man happily declares himself to be a feminist. In 2014, when *Elle* magazine published photographs of political leaders and celebrities wearing 'This is what a feminist looks like' t-shirts, the powerful men in them were applauded. Of course, any celebration of feminism is welcome, and there is no doubt that woman abuse has moved higher up the political and social agenda since I wrote the first edition of this book. However, society's misogyny is much more subtle and insidious than a slogan on a t-shirt; we must ask ourselves what, for all the concerned posturing, has actually changed. If society really has changed and feminism is no longer a dirty word, why are such huge numbers of women still being brutalised and killed?

## Society's response

Clearly, some progress has been made. For example, there are now more specialist services for abused women and children. When I wrote the first edition of this book, no one had ever heard of an Independent Domestic Violence Advocate (IDVA). And yet now there are hundreds of these specialist workers across the UK. Based in hospitals, the courts and the community, IDVAs support women and children at the very highest risk of serious injury or death. They often work in police stations in order to provide immediate support to women and the officers involved in their cases. There are now also culturally specific services for women and children from black, Asian and specific minority ethnic communities, although, as mentioned previously, these are often desperately underfunded.

There is still an issue of scale. More than one million women experience domestic abuse every year; England and Wales have nowhere near enough service provision to support them all. What about all the women who never receive the specialist support they need? What about the women who try to flee their violent partner but find that there is no refuge space available to them? Perhaps the police might arrest and charge the perpetrator, one might think, so he can no longer harm her. The police receive a domestic violence-related call every 30 seconds[36] – yet all too often, no arrest is made.

A strong police response can deliver a clear message: to abusive men, that assaulting a woman is a criminal offence and there will be consequences; to abused women, that they do not have to put up with abusive behaviour; and to society, that such behaviour is criminal and should not be tolerated. Yet 25 years after I wrote about the negative attitudes of the police in the first edition of this book, their response to domestic violence remains inadequate – and in some cases, as I have already highlighted through the tragic case of Sabina Akhtar, potentially fatal.

There has been some improvement in the police response. Almost all police forces now have specialist units to deal with domestic violence and there has been a cultural shift in the way the crime is viewed. Police officers now *know* they cannot ignore domestic violence – if only because they want to avoid getting into trouble. Some forces have introduced specialist domestic violence training for officers, so they understand how to respond to abused women. However, there is still a long way to go before all women get the protection they deserve.

This fact was highlighted in October 2013, when the then Home Secretary, Theresa May, asked Her Majesty's Inspectorate of Constabulary (HMIC) – the body that oversees police performance in the UK – to conduct a six-month inspection into how well police forces were responding to victims of domestic violence.

The final report came to a damning conclusion, finding that 'the overall police response to victims of domestic abuse is not good enough'.[37] HMIC found 'unacceptable failings in core policing activities'. The report showed that officers were failing to collect evidence and arrest violent men. It also revealed deeply entrenched problems with police culture and attitudes towards victims, with many officers failing to take domestic violence seriously or even believe women when they report abuse. It found that officers were often dismissive and judgemental of women and made them feel that *they* were to blame for the abuse. Officers simply weren't listening to women – and instead listened to their abusers. Every day, I would – and still do – hear stories from women whose experiences highlight these failings. But HMIC's report meant policy-makers finally began listening.

When I was working in the refuges, I heard countless horrific stories of poor police response. One woman told me how she escaped from her husband, who had attacked her with a chisel. She ran into the street, with her child in her arms, with blood streaming down her face. As she did so she spotted a police car, and with relief flagged it down. When she told the two male officers that it was her husband who had inflicted her injuries, they told her there was nothing they could do, and drove off. Her case was never investigated.

Another woman, a widow in her sixties, met a man she wanted to marry. Then one night he attacked her, ripping a hank of hair from her head and knocking her out by slamming her head against a table. On leaving hospital, she asked the police to take action. When they heard it was her fiancé who had attacked her, they were indifferent. It was only after seven months of lobbying and complaining that she finally secured an arrest. Hazel told me that, on one of the numerous occasions when she called the police, she was frightened and hysterical, which prompted one of the officers to tell her, 'Calm down, or we'll put you away.'

Another woman told me that while she was separated from her violent husband he turned up hammering at the door and threatening her. She was terrified – she tried to phone her father on the landline, but discovered that her husband had got in earlier and broken the handset. 'I thought, "I'm trapped. I can't get out of the balcony. I can't jump one floor. I can't phone anybody to tell them,"' she told me. 'So I kept the children in the living room and kept them quiet and I was looking out of the kitchen window, which is away from the street-door landing, and I happened to see a neighbour. I only knew him to say hello to, but I shouted down, "Excuse me, please ring the police – my husband's a bit violent. Please, please ring the police."

'I felt so low to have to swallow my pride and let somebody know what was happening to me. I thought, He'll go upstairs and think, "Stupid person, she's a bit mad, shouting out of the window that her husband's attacking her" – but he did call the police. My husband was shouting, "You slag, you whore, who have you got in there?" and I heard the police coming so I opened the door. They took him away, but I discovered later that they didn't take him to the police station; they dropped him off around the corner at his local pub. He told me later, "Oh, the police were great. They said, 'Look, just play along with us, jump in the car. Where's your local?'" And they dropped him off outside.'

Another time, he pounced out of the blue, while she was returning from the shops pushing her baby in her pram, with her son walking alongside. 'I thought I was safe in the street,' she said. 'I thought, "He wouldn't start in the street." Then: slap, punch around the face with the back of his hand. He grabbed the pram, and I wouldn't let go, and I said no, and I was crying. With that he hit me so hard I let go of the pram, and he ran off with the baby. I thought, "What do I do? My baby – he's got my baby – he's violent – is he going to hit her?" So I phoned the police. He'd taken her to his brother's. I ran round there and the police turned up.

'Apparently I just screamed, I was in such a state – I wanted my daughter back, and they just said, "There's nothing you can do. She's in safe hands, she's with your husband, and the house is clean and everything. Promise us that you'll leave it alone and you won't come back." I said yes, but I was in such a state, I wanted my daughter back, so I went back, and begged him through the door. All of a sudden the police turned up and said, "Look, if you don't go back, you're going to be arrested." I said, "What for? I'm doing nothing wrong in wanting my daughter back," and they arrested me.

'The most humiliating thing was going into the police station, having to take my wedding ring off, my clips out of my hair, as if I was going to do something drastic. They wouldn't allow me to smoke, and I had to turn out my shopping bags. One was really nasty as if I was a criminal – I felt like I'd mugged an old lady. They said, "We won't keep you – you're going to go to court in the morning," and I thought, "I've never been to court in my life. Why are they doing this to me?" I was petrified, because I didn't know what it would involve. The judge was awful...I was bound over to keep the peace for two years.

'The police arrested *me*,' said the woman incredulously, 'yet they dropped *him* off round the corner at the pub.'

These cases happened many years ago, but the dismissals and negative attitudes persist today. When women report domestic abuse, police officers still tell them not to bother. 'If you press charges, he's only going to be charged with criminal damage,' they say. Or, 'Going to court will mean a lot of stress for you.'

It sometimes seems that police are most concerned with women they see as 'genuine victims' – those who fit neatly into their definition of what an abused woman should be, rather than women who may also have been prostitutes, or who have drink or drug problems. In 2015, two police officers in the West Midlands admitted to inadvertently leaving an abusive voicemail on an alleged domestic violence victim's phone, calling her a 'f***ing slag' and a 'bitch'.[38] Even worse, a 2016 HMIC report into abuse of power by police for sexual gain found that 39 per cent of the allegations involved victims of domestic abuse.[39] It is horrific but unsurprising. How can women be expected to report their abuse, when the people they should be able to trust to protect them may actually abuse them all over again? Perhaps that is one of the reasons why it is estimated that only 24 per cent of women ever report their abuse to the police.[40]

Then there are things that really should be common sense. Providing a translator, for example, so that a woman's sister-in-law is not left to translate the abuse her brother has inflicted, as happened in one recent case. Or questioning a woman about what happened away from her perpetrator.

The first response officer does not always see the bigger picture or understand the context – the pattern of intimidation and abuse that escalates over time. The officer only sees the broken phone, the threatening text or the slashed tyre. Very often, mistakes are made because officers do not understand the power imbalance of the relationship. They may not understand that a man might be minimising his abuse in order to get away with it; or that a woman may be so frightened, so controlled, that she does not reveal the whole truth.

For decades I have been listening to police officers telling me that the real problem is the women. They just don't report. They withdraw their support. They change their story. They don't turn up at court. They even go back to the perpetrator. But women tell me the other side of the story.

Often – even if a woman is willing and able to support a prosecution, she is told that there is no police officer available to take a statement after all. One woman I spoke to – in hospital, recovering from a brutal assault – wasn't at home when the police called round to take a statement, so she tried to follow up when she was discharged. But she was told it was too late – the police couldn't wait around forever.

Sometimes the police fail to take photographic evidence – perhaps there wasn't a camera free. Or the photographs didn't come out right and couldn't be used after all. Or they have lost the photographs of her injuries and the injuries have now faded.

These negative experiences leave severe and lasting impressions on women. They learn very quickly that even if a man beats, rapes and strangles his partner he might just get away with it.

I know there are many dedicated police officers who are working hard to change things. There *are* solutions, and when police officers take the right approach the results can save lives. One woman I supported felt much safer when the police put extra flags on her address and gave her a panic alarm and a fireproof letterbox. Another woman, who was returning from abroad having tried to escape her violent husband, was met by a police officer on the aeroplane. The police officer helped her and her children leave the airport through a staff exit so they would not be found in the arrivals area, and then drove them to a refuge.

Going the extra mile for an abused woman, listening to her and respecting her, understanding the reality of her experiences...This is what increases a woman's confidence in the police. This is what keeps her safe.

Too often, however, this is not what happens – and the consequences can be fatal. In recent years I have worked closely with a number of families who have lost loved ones to domestic violence in situations where the police – or other state agencies – failed to protect them. These families have endured unimaginable pain: the pain of losing a loved one to violence, compounded by the pain of knowing that the death might have been prevented.

### The ultimate failing

In 2010, Rachael Slack and her toddler, Auden, were stabbed to death by Rachael's ex-partner, Andrew Cairns. Rachael was pregnant at the time. Rachael reported to the police that Andrew had threatened to kill her and take Auden. Andrew's neighbour had separately reported that he had threatened to 'grab' Auden. Andrew's mental state was also assessed by a number of medical professionals in the days and weeks leading up to the killing. Although police arrested Andrew, he was released on bail and five days later he killed Rachael and Auden. It was revealed at an inquest in 2013 that the police had assessed Rachael and Auden as being at high risk of serious harm or homicide – but they did not warn Rachael so that she could take steps to protect herself, her son and her unborn baby. The inquest found that failures by Derbyshire Police 'more than minimally contributed' to Rachael and Auden's deaths. Rachael's brother Hayden and his wife Melony have worked with Refuge in order to raise awareness of domestic violence and the police response so that other families might be spared their grief. I remember speaking to Melony on what would have been Rachael's 42nd birthday. 'We would have been swapping stories about her fabulous and fun 40th birthday party and reflecting on how Auden had coped with his first half-term at school,' she said. 'Perhaps we would have been laughing as we watched Auden run around and play with his little brother and listened to Rachael's plans for his third birthday in November. From time to time the festivities would be punctuated by Rachael's unique, infectious laugh and she would have almost certainly been jollying her mum along.' Andrew Cairns denied Auden, Rachael and her unborn baby this life – but avoidable failings by the police also played their part.

The family of Maria Stubbings also lives with the knowledge that more could have been done to save her life. Maria was strangled with a dog lead by her ex-partner, Marc Chivers, in 2008. Marc was already known to police, having recently been released from jail for killing another woman. In July Maria reported that Marc had assaulted her. She was assessed as 'high risk' and was given a panic alarm, but this was taken away a day later when Marc was arrested. Later that year he was found guilty of assault but was released immediately as he had already spent time in jail on remand, awaiting trial. Nobody told Maria he was now a free man. That December, Maria repeatedly begged the police for help, but they failed to take her seriously. Officers eventually attended her home, but Marc answered the door and told them Maria was away. The officers took no steps against Marc and did not search the property. Instead they left a calling card and asked Marc to inform Maria that they had called. Maria's body was found the next day. An investigation by the Independent Police Complaints Commission (IPCC) showed that serious police failures by Essex Police meant Maria was not afforded the protection she deserved. At the inquest, the jury found that the force had made a catalogue of errors and had failed in almost every part of its investigation. As Celia Peachey, Maria's daughter, said to me: 'My mum was not a statistic – she was a person. She had a right to protection and she was denied that basic human right. I truly believe that she would still be alive today if the police had done their jobs properly.'

Six years after Maria's murder, the Government began a national roll-out of the domestic violence disclosure scheme. Named 'Clare's Law', after Clare Wood, who was murdered by her ex-boyfriend in 2009, the scheme allows police to disclose information on request about a partner's previous history of domestic violence or violent acts. Clare's Law sounds good on paper, but in reality it will do very little to help the hundreds of thousands of women and children who experience domestic violence. The vast majority of perpetrators are never known to the police. If a woman enquires about her partner under Clare's Law, she may be told that he has no history of violence and then believe that she is safe, when this may not be the case. And what will happen if a woman is told that her partner has a history of violence? Will she be expected to pack her bags and leave straight away? As we know, it is not that simple.

Cassie Hasanovic – a young mother of two – might also have been saved if the police and Crown Prosecution Service had taken appropriate steps. Cassie was killed by her estranged husband, Hajrudin Hasanovic, as she was getting into a car to go to a refuge, in front of her children and her mother. Like Rachael, Cassie had been assessed by police as being at high risk of serious harm after she repeatedly reported her concerns and following an assault by Hajrudin. On the morning of her death, Cassie had decided to go to a refuge because she knew it was not safe to stay in her home. She begged police to escort her to the refuge. They refused. The jury at the inquest in Chichester returned a verdict of unlawful killing and criticised the Crown Prosecution Service and Sussex Police for failing to take steps to safeguard her life. 'Cassie was a beautiful, courageous young woman who did everything within her power to protect herself and her children,' Cassie's mother, Sharon de Souza, said. 'She was a wonderful mother whose greatest wish was to watch her children grow up.'

Christine Lee and her daughter, Lucy Lee, were shot dead by Christine's ex-partner, John Lowe, at his puppy farm in Surrey in February 2014. Christine's other daughter, Stacy, has been threatened by John and she had reported him, repeatedly, to Surrey Police. Although the police removed John's guns, they later returned them to him. After the murders, Surrey Police apologised to Stacy for returning the guns after they were confiscated; but at the time of writing, Stacy is still waiting for the IPCC to publish its findings.

Even if the police are sympathetic and take woman abuse seriously, the number of men who go scot-free when they have inflicted the most brutal injuries on the women they live with is alarming. Getting a positive police response is often a postcode lottery. Frequently, the police do not arrest – or it takes great persuasion for them to treat assaults seriously and take action. And remember, domestic violence is a crime where there is rarely doubt over who the perpetrator is – these aren't burglars who have broken in with masks; they are husbands and boyfriends. Often, victims are not informed on how their complaint has been dealt with – they live in fear, not knowing whether their abuser has been arrested or released on bail, or whether their case has been stamped with 'No Further Action'. For a woman who has been terrorised in her own home for months or even years, imagine the fear this limbo creates.

Such problems extend to the criminal court. Take restraining orders. Handed down by judges, these pieces of paper forbid a perpetrator from contacting or going within a certain distance of his victim, either for a set or indefinite period of time. The penalty for breaching a restraining order can be up to five years in prison. Prior to this measure, a woman could leave the court room and have her perpetrator follow her down the street, even if he had been convicted. But restraining orders only improve lives if they are used effectively. Sometimes, women never receive the paperwork. Sometimes, the police do not. Sometimes, the Crown Prosecution Service simply forgets to issue the papers. That means that if a woman phones to say her abuser is outside her house, breaking his order, there is no record of it. The correct tool exists, but the systems to enact it are poor and women frequently fall through the gaps.

One husband followed his wife to a refuge at midnight and was banging on the door, threatening to kill her. She was so terrified that the doctors gave her tranquillisers. She had obtained an injunction, with powers of arrest, so that in such a situation the police could step in immediately. They did so, but instead of being held overnight and taken to court the next morning to be dealt with (which was the purpose of the injunction), he was released after five hours. He came straight back to the refuge and resumed his threats. The examples I could include on this subject would go on for pages and pages.

Then there is the battle to get perpetrators prosecuted for their abuse. Figures from the Crown Prosecution Service show that the number of prosecutions and convictions for domestic abuse is increasing year on year; this is thanks, in no small part, to two consecutive Directors of Public Prosecution who have viewed violence against women as a priority. Yet the figures are a drop in the ocean when we consider the number of women experiencing abuse. In 2015–16, there was a 75 per cent conviction rate for domestic abuse[41] but we must remember that this only takes into consideration the cases that the CPS decides to prosecute. The overwhelming majority of cases are not prosecuted. So very few incidents that are reported to police (fewer than 10 per cent) will result in conviction. The Crown Prosecution Service frequently decides that there is insufficient evidence to prosecute, or it might downgrade crimes in order to make prosecution easier. It is also concerning that recently there has been a reduction in referrals from the police to the Crown Prosecution Service for domestic abuse crimes.[42]

Instead of pushing for prosecutions to help reduce the cases of woman abuse, the authorities stack the odds against a woman. In one case, the Crown Prosecutor turned to an abused woman, who was armed with perfectly adequate evidence against her partner, and suggested, 'This case is going to be very stressful for you. Do you think you ought to change your mind?' Having gone through so much to actually arrive at this stage of proceedings, the woman was so worried by his comments that she was persuaded to drop the case. The Crown Prosecutor may have been genuinely concerned for her feelings – but the result was that her abuser walked away, free. The court had simply carried on where the husband had left off, undermining her courage and confidence. I cannot imagine the prosecutor would have said the same to the victim of a burglary.

Sometimes, even if the case does get to court, women tell me they wait months and months for the hearing. Sometimes they are told to go to the wrong court. Or the court room is double-booked because the court has assumed – with it being a domestic violence case – that the victim probably won't show up.

In most cases it is hard enough for the woman to go ahead with a prosecution as it is – her partner may be threatening her, and agencies may be putting pressure on her to keep the family unit intact – without her feeling that she has no real support in court either.

It is this lack of support that is often to blame for a woman faltering at the final hurdle, at a time when she is usually being intimidated by her partner and is trying to cope with a whole set of emotions, such as fear of the future, guilt and shame – a time when she is most in need of encouragement.

When there is a successful prosecution – and a guilty verdict – women are often disappointed with the sentencing. Still, custodial sentences – even for the most serious cases of Actual Bodily Harm (ABH) – are rare. A woman can be beaten black and blue, left with broken bones and slashes and cuts, and still her partner can walk away from court a free man. The threshold for an incident to be 'Grievous Bodily Harm' (GBH) is extremely high. A harrowing BBC documentary[43] highlighted the trial of Paul Hopkins, who assaulted his partner Sabrina, in April 2015. In the documentary, Sabrina says of the attack: 'I've never been so frightened – I honestly thought I was going to die. I thought he was going to kill me. If the police hadn't have come when they did he would have done. He was still going then. I can't even begin to explain what it felt like…it's almost resigning yourself to the fact that "this is it, I'm going to die. I am going to die." Then I got to the point while he was beating where it was like: "Please, this next punch, just let this be the last one so he kills me and it stops, so I won't feel it anymore."' Paul was arrested and charged with GBH with intent, and remanded in custody. Later, Paul pleaded guilty to a reduced charge of ABH. The Crown Prosecutor assured the police it was the worst case of ABH she had ever seen – yet Paul was only given two years in jail. In reality, he is likely to serve half – and because he spent time on remand, he will spend even less time behind bars.[44]

Agencies other than the police, though meaning well, often fail abused women, too. Blaming the woman is such an easy trap to fall into that even counsellors sometimes make the mistake of asking, 'What did you do to make him hit you?' All this does is heighten the woman's self-doubt, guilt and shame, and imply that the man is in some way entitled to be violent. Her partner will almost certainly have brainwashed her into believing that she is at least partly responsible for his behaviour – now here is her counsellor reinforcing that view. Often counsellors insist on seeing both the man and the woman together, inevitably making it difficult for the woman to speak freely and implying that the man is not entirely to blame.

'Are you depriving him of sex?' 'What did you do to upset him?' 'Did you start it?' are all loaded questions which women seeking help encounter all the time, from the kindest people. One woman told me that the response from her neighbour was: 'Perhaps you should pay more attention to him.' Other women tell me that counsellors have made suggestions like: 'Perhaps you could make yourself a little more attractive.'

One physically battered woman whose husband was persuaded to have therapy told me: 'The therapist said I should treat him as a toddler, as if he had just found his feet, and just found his anger, and he was experiencing it for the first time, and that he had to express that, but gradually things would calm down and we would have a much more fulfilling, expressive relationship.' As this woman wryly pointed out, 'What she wasn't aware of is how terrifying it is to live with a man who is six feet tall, weighs 12 stone and is an expert in karate, who "behaves like a toddler" and flies off into inexplicable rages at any time.'

All these responses shift the blame onto the woman, and suggest that the remedy lies with *her* rather than the abuser. If he is not held to account for his behaviour, then we give him permission to continue.

Some women tell me how they have been rushed to casualty units with wounds inflicted by their partners – only for their abusers to be allowed into the units with them, where they frequently tell the medical staff their own versions of the story and are invariably believed. Other women have gone to their general practitioners in desperation, only to be given tranquillisers by doctors too busy to ask enough questions. Others have turned to the Church, only to be reminded about the sanctity of marriage and asked, 'Perhaps you are not being attentive and caring enough as a wife?'

Even the language we use implies that the woman must take her share of the blame. Instead of talking about 'woman abuse' we say 'domestic violence', 'conjugal violence' and 'abusive relationships'. Even if the woman is not blamed exclusively, the usual attitude is that she must share the guilt. 'It takes two' is such a hackneyed phrase that people never even stop to think whether it might have any foundation in truth.

Society is locked into the idea that if a woman is abused she is somehow responsible. Blaming the woman is almost instinctive. 'She probably deserved it,' people say, with no real knowledge of the facts, 'and anyway he only slapped her the once.' Or 'She shouldn't have gone on and on at him', or 'If she were my wife, I'd have done the same thing.' Even people who are genuinely concerned to help the woman fall into the trap of diverting the blame in her direction: 'You chose him – you'll have to make the best of it.' 'He seems such a nice chap – it can't be all his fault.' 'Perhaps you both need help.' All these phrases are regularly trotted out to women by people who mean well, yet unwittingly put the onus on the woman.

Well-meaning people often practise amateur marriage counselling but invariably they try to repair the relationship rather than make the man own up to his behaviour. Very rarely does anyone tell the woman – or the man – the most important thing they both need to know: that *she* is not responsible for her abuser's behaviour. No woman can *make* a man abuse her. It is a choice *he* makes. The upshot of all this woman-blaming is inevitably that *she* believes it too (after all, women are part of the same society), making it even easier for an abuser to excuse himself.

The blaming, the passing of the buck, the denial, the excuses and the justifications go on and on, round and round in a vicious circle. While women continue to suffer, men fail to take responsibility for their behaviour and our society turns a sceptical face towards the women it should be helping, preferring to believe the popular myths about woman abuse, rather than look for deeper truths which may be harder to tackle.

Instead of looking boldly in the mirror, we allow ourselves to be distracted by myths.

# Myths

'He was just drunk', 'He was jealous', 'He's having a hard time at work', 'He comes from a violent home' – these are the kinds of excuses I hear repeatedly when people talk about cases of men abusing women. Even more incredibly, people have asked me, 'Is it true that pollution is a cause of wife abuse?' One man even said to me, 'I hear wife abuse is on the increase because of the disastrous England football results.'

Some factors such as drink and jealousy may contribute to the abuse of women, but I do not believe that any actually *cause* it. And, what is more worrying, the tendency to write off abusive behaviour as just the result of one drink too many, unemployment or a jealous rage can actually perpetuate such abuse, because while society accepts these excuses no one feels obliged to look for the real root cause and do something about it.

I believe the reasons why men abuse women are much more complex, but before we discuss them it is important to cut through some of the myths which obscure the real causes.

### *'Some women are turned on by violence'*

There is a whole school of thought which maintains that women secretly enjoy being abused – in fact they are attracted to it. Some people go one step further in putting forward a theory which, I feel, has perpetuated the idea that women are to blame. They believe that some women are 'chemically addicted' to violence[45] – that some imbalance in their chemical make-up draws them towards pain.

For a start there is no medical evidence whatsoever to support this theory of chemical addiction. And the theory does not explain why men batter women. Even if this theory were correct, there would still have to be men out there prepared to abuse such women and satisfy their 'craving'. Such women could not *cause* men to be violent, only the men could make that choice. To suggest that a woman could turn a gentle, considerate man into someone who controls, subjugates and humiliates her is quite ludicrous.

Furthermore, in my experience, women usually have no way of knowing that they are embarking on a life with an abusive man. Remember the stories of our six women? When they met their partners, they each thought they had found a soul mate who was charming, gentle, kind and considerate. They had not yet discovered the abusive side to these men's characters. How could they be attracted, or addicted, to violence they were not even aware of?

I am not denying that there are masochistic women – any more than that there are masochistic men – but this has no bearing on woman abuse. If abused women were really masochistic, if they were really attracted to the abuse, would they come to Refuge for help? It simply does not make sense.

The assumption that abused women must be masochistic or chemically addicted to violence has largely arisen because many women find it difficult to leave their abusers. If they stay, the argument goes, they must like it. However, many do leave. And if they stay, as the women I have interviewed explained so graphically in the previous chapters, it is because they are trapped, and because society tells them they are worthless without a man – not because they are masochists or chemically addicted.

## 'What about abused men?'

One of the easiest ways of avoiding an issue is to turn it on its head. So when many people are asked to face the problem of woman abuse, they insist that it is a one-sided question, that men are as abused as women. For some reason, people seem to think that if they can show that men are abused too, then woman abuse is not a problem they have to think about. It seems that woman abuse is the one crime where people instinctively leap to the defence of the offender.

Refuge does support a small number of men who have experienced domestic and sexual violence, through outreach programmes and independent advocacy services. Nobody, whatever their gender or sexuality, should have to live in fear of violence and abuse. However, the evidence shows that, overwhelmingly, domestic violence is a male prerogative: four times as many women as men are killed by their current or former partners. Despite the fact that women are three times more likely to be arrested for incidents of abuse,[46] Crown Prosecution Service data shows that 93 per cent of defendants in domestic abuse court cases are male, and 84 per cent of victims are female.[47]

We know from research that the intensity and severity of violence used by men against women is more extreme and more likely to include physical violence, threats and harassment.[48] Female victims of domestic violence experience more serious psychological consequences than male victims and are much more likely to feel afraid of their partners.[49]

Generally speaking, men are stronger than women, and can inflict much worse injuries – particularly when a woman is pregnant, and there are then two casualties.

As far as emotional abuse is concerned, everyone must be familiar with that popular caricature of the nagging wife, shrieking at her poor downtrodden husband – the butt of music-hall jokes, literature and popular songs. Why is it always women who seem to be tagged with negative labels? Why doesn't anyone say, 'What about nagging men?' After all, abusive men constantly nag, harass and criticise their partners. And abused women, contrary to the stereotype, do everything they can to avoid 'nagging' – because they are afraid of provoking more abuse.

I will not deny for a moment that a woman who does nothing but nag and criticise is unattractive and irritating. But however bitingly sarcastic, however cruel and venomous a woman may be, I do not believe that a man feels that he is being *controlled* by such a woman in the way that a woman is controlled by her abuser. Nor is he trapped in the same way. Men who are unhappy in their relationships may stay with their partners for the sake of the children, or because their lives are predictable, if unexciting. But they do not stay because they are trapped by insurmountable social and emotional barriers. They do not have to face the problem of trying to find good, well-paid jobs after years of rearing children. When it comes to leaving, women have far fewer options than men.

Woman abuse is part of a worldwide pattern of gender inequality and oppression. The abuse of men by their female partners is unacceptable but it is not sanctioned and encouraged in the same way woman abuse is. We do victims of both sexes a disservice by suggesting that what they experience is the same.

The bottom line is that men do not feel controlled and trapped by their partners in the way that women in abusive situations do.

## 'She provoked it – she deserved whatever she got'

It simply is not true that the abuse most women suffer is in any way provoked by them. As we have seen, many women are attacked when they are asleep. Laura was sexually abused while she was asleep. Hazel was sitting quietly smoking a cigarette when Jimmy snatched the cigarette from her hand and pulled out a lock of her hair. One epileptic woman was dragged out of her wheelchair by her husband, who walked through the door and said, 'What are you sitting there like that for?' She had done nothing, said nothing. He simply attacked her. There may be no row – nothing that a woman can put her finger on, which causes the abuse.

If a woman is particularly unpleasant, do we say a burglar is entitled to rob her home? However appallingly a woman may behave, this does not excuse abuse. A man still has a choice. He does not have to use violence, he does not have to be verbally or emotionally abusive. Frustrated as he may be, he can learn to control his anger, to walk away, to try to resolve the problem with his partner calmly, to accept that she has a right to her own point of view.

## 'It only happens in low-income families'

That could not be further from the truth. Abusers and abused women come from all income brackets, classes and creeds – as I mentioned in Chapter 1. Remember Joel Steinberg and Hedda Nussbaum, Charlotte and John Fedders, Sheryl Gascoigne, Ulrika Jonsson, Rihanna, the late Lynda Bellingham and the other famous names you have read about in the press and heard about on the television.

I constantly receive phone calls from women who are married to wealthy and influential abusers, and many come to me for advice. It may be that they do not always figure in the statistics, because they do not necessarily move into refuges or contact the police for help.

## 'It's because he grew up in a violent home'

Many people believe that boys who grow up in violent homes will repeat the pattern as adults. Yet studies exploring the link between exposure to domestic violence in childhood and a domestically violent adulthood reveal mixed results. Most suggest that the majority of children who are exposed do not repeat this behaviour in later relationships.[50] Personally I would say that while it is true that many boys who experience abuse grow up to be abusers, some turn their backs on all forms of abuse in revulsion against their childhood experiences. Growing up in an abusive home may be a factor, but it cannot be the sole cause – otherwise all men who grew up in these circumstances would go on to abuse women.

Yes, boys in such homes do receive messages that they should be aggressive, powerful, in control, but the family is only a microcosm of society. These messages are everywhere in children's books, on TV adverts, in magazines, in lyrics to popular music and in videogames. Boys are given the impression very early on in life that women do not deserve respect.

The family may be a great influence – but that family is only behaving in the way that some families have behaved for generations, because our society has grown up with the idea that men are supposed to keep 'their women' in line, even to the point of being violent and abusive.

## 'There's a pattern of abuse in her family'

The argument is that there are women who, though they may not be chemically addicted to violence, choose violent men – sometimes again and again – because they have grown up in abusive homes and have not developed any self-esteem. If their mothers are passive, they behave the same way. Also, the argument goes, such women have only known abusive behaviour. So, subconsciously, they feel comfortable with it. It is 'normal' and familiar to them. Men who treat them well seem unexciting and tedious.

There is simply no correlation between a woman's background and the chances of her becoming an abused woman. Having met thousands of abused women, I know that many women who grow up in loving families find themselves involved with abusive partners as adults. Hazel told me that when she met Jimmy she was hoping to find the kind of happiness her parents had enjoyed. Moreover, in my experience the last thing women do is seek out abusive men. And, as we know, Charm Syndrome Man never reveals himself in his true colours at the beginning of the relationship. So how could the women know they had 'found' an abuser?

Nor does this theory explain why men abuse women. Even if there were women running around, desperately looking for abusive men, they could not turn men who have no abusive tendencies into abusers, just to suit them.

It *is* possible that some women from abusive backgrounds end up with abusive men, but given that one in four women will be abused at some point in their lives it is hardly surprising. Nor is it surprising that some women leave their abusers only to end up with someone else who treats them just as badly. Almost every woman could find herself involved with an abusive man – whatever her background or emotional make-up.

After all, he and his partner are still part of a patriarchal society, a society which nourishes woman abuse. Instead of asking 'Why does she choose another violent man?', we should be asking 'Why does he find another woman to batter?'

### 'He must be sick'

Very often, people's instinctive reaction when they hear of a man abusing his partner is: he must be crazy, or he must be socially or sexually inadequate (one abused woman, married to a journalist, said to me, 'Surely there must be an organic base to his problem?'). These are understandable reactions, since to accept that the man is not sick, that he is just Mr Average, is an idea that most people – particularly women – find extremely disturbing, since if it is true, all women run the risk of finding themselves living with an abuser.

Unfortunately, it *is* true. Of course some men who batter their partners are indeed clinically sick, but the majority are not. Many are highly respected, competent, perfectly functioning figures, such as judges, journalists and doctors. Research shows that the proportion of abusers who are mentally unbalanced is no higher than in society as a whole. Furthermore, if these men are mentally ill, why don't they abuse their employers or strangers in the street? Why is it only their partners, or occasionally a relative who is so close to the woman as to be seen almost as an extension of her? In addition, there are many men who are clinically sick, impotent or socially inadequate and who do not abuse women.

### 'He has criminal tendencies anyway'

Some men who abuse their partners have histories of violence or criminal records. However, for the majority of women I have counselled, their violent partners are perfectly law-abiding in their public lives; it is only behind closed doors that their violence is played out.

### 'He must be drunk or on drugs'

It is true that some men who abuse their partners are drug-takers or alcoholics, but this is in no way universal – nor can it be blamed for the abuse.

Many of the women I talk to live with men who drink too much and then assault them, but they also assault them when they are sober. Women tell me they take extra precautions if they know their partners have been drinking, because they know it gives the men an excuse to be more aggressive. But the alcohol is not the root cause.

Blaming drink or drugs is a way of denying responsibility by pleading loss of control. It is easy for a man to say, 'I was out of control – I was drunk,' or 'I don't remember – I was high at the time,' and society will accept the excuse. But such a man is in control enough to hit only his partner – not others – and he is usually in control enough to stop short of killing the woman.

Most men who batter their wives do not have drink problems at all, and have never taken drugs. Conversely, many men drink too much or take drugs, but would never abuse their partners.

Blaming drink or drugs is simply an excuse. It dodges the real issue. After all, if abuse is simply a product of alcohol or drugs, why don't women who drink or take drugs batter men in equal numbers?

### 'He was just jealous'

As we have seen, Charm Syndrome Man is usually very jealous indeed – but we must remind ourselves why he is jealous. He is jealous because he cannot bear the idea of losing *control*. He sees his partner as a possession, and no one but him must get close to her. Many men see it as macho to behave in this fashion. People frequently say, 'He's jealous because he's insecure' – and this is partly true. He *is* insecure, because he is frightened of losing his 'possession'. Besides, many men are insecure and jealous, yet they do not feel entitled to abuse their partners because of it.

Jealousy is only one facet of an abuser's controlling behaviour, but it is one of the excuses most readily accepted by abused women and society – and because of its romantic implications it is the one most easily exploited by Charm Syndrome Man. Invariably *he* ends up with the sympathy – not the woman, whose partner interrogates her until the early hours, forbids her to see her friends, or beats her senseless for some imagined misdemeanour.

Jealousy may be a contributory factor in the abuse of women, certainly, but it is not the root cause.

### 'They just have unmet dependency needs'

Many psychologists argue that both the abuser and his partner are dependent on each other. This dependency is created at infancy, when the child is nourished, encouraged, loved and protected by its mother, and feels panicky and insecure when ignored. For both men and women, the argument goes, this need for someone to fill the mother role lingers in adulthood, so that they both believe they cannot survive without each other, they rely on each other to fulfil every emotional need. When an abusive man believes that his partner is not satisfying these needs, or fears that she might be about to abandon him, he becomes violent or emotionally abusive, while the woman, in her belief that they are vital to each other, feels she cannot leave.

I am not dismissing this theory, but it is only a part of the picture. Many people have 'unmet dependency needs', but they do not become abusers, or find themselves living with abusers. Instead they may withdraw, or eat too much, underperform at work or become workaholics.

The theory is flawed – because if all babies are brought up with these needs, why is it only the males who become abusers? And the theory fails to take into account the social pressures and lack of facilities which prevent women from leaving their abusers. Nor does it encompass any of the ways in which men are encouraged to batter and abuse by a society which does not take them to task. And if all men and women have these dependency needs, why is it only some men abuse, that only some women are abused? And what about the influence of fathers?

## 'He is under stress'

I hear this one over and over again. Certainly, some men who abuse their wives are suffering from stress but, again, this is an excuse, not a cause. Many men who are stressed do not abuse their wives: similarly, many men who abuse their wives cannot claim to be under stress.

Women also suffer from stress. They may have jobs which demand a great deal of responsibility and decision-making, they too may be made redundant, or they may be trying to care for elderly relatives or look after their family, with an abusive and controlling husband who beats them and refuses to give them money for the housekeeping – yet women rarely beat or abuse their partners to the extent that men abuse women. Stress is simply a red herring.

## 'He just loses his temper sometimes'

Many people argue that an abusive man merely loses his temper. He is out of control, or, as Deborah Sinclair suggests in *Understanding Wife Assault*, he has 'poor impulse control', he is a 'walking time-bomb' which suddenly explodes.[51]

I would argue that, on the contrary, consciously or subconsciously, an abuser is very much in control. You have only to listen to the stories of abused women to realise that these men are very selective in their violence. Hazel told me that even when Jimmy was trying to choke her, 'He seemed out of control in one way, but there was something controlling this "out of control" part. Even when he appeared to be acting wildly, he was aware of what he was doing.'

Like many abusers, he rarely left marks on prominent parts of her body, since that would attract the attention of friends and neighbours. 'When we were first married,' she noted, 'he broke my nose twice, but later on he started hitting me on the body, because it didn't show. When he hit my face, it got marked, and I lost a lot of jobs because I couldn't show up with my face all marked. So after a while he learned that I couldn't go to work if my face was marked.' Jimmy was no fool: he was unemployed, and his wife was the sole wage-earner.

Laura, too, noticed that her husband learned by his mistakes, and she was frightened that his violence could be so calculated. 'In the beginning,' she says, echoing Hazel's story, 'the first times he hit me, it was a regular black eye, but after that I'm quite sure he took care that it wasn't anywhere that was going to show. I always felt that it was controlled too; and that he could, if he wanted to, hurt me much more. He hit me enough for it to hurt, but not to show; which is pretty frightening, because it's a controlled kind of violence, rather than saying he was drunk out of his head and didn't know what he was doing.'

James was selective about when and where he hit Laura – until the last time. 'He would hit me behind a closed door at the bottom of the house so the children wouldn't wake up,' she says. 'He knew that if the children ever became involved, that would give me the strength to leave.' On one occasion, he even stopped hitting her, telling her to make a cup of tea, then started again once he had drunk it.

Abusive men are also selective in that they will destroy a woman's possessions, but not their own. They will not smash the television if they enjoy watching it. They do not beat up their bosses or people they hold in high esteem and do not want to alienate – because that would not be to their advantage.

Immediately after an abuser has acted violently towards his partner, or if he is interrupted during his assault, he is frequently able to turn on the charm to convince neighbours, friends and police that the woman is exaggerating things – that he would not dream of laying a finger on her. Does this sound like a man who is out of control?

Anger is something which *can* be controlled. If you were to make somebody stand on the edge of a cliff and say to them, 'If you lose your temper, I'll push you off', that person would almost certainly manage to keep control. The same is true of abusive men. They *choose* to use their temper as a controlling device. Some are ice cool in planning their attacks, and are therefore particularly frightening. Others less so. Yet even an abuser who seems to be out of control and acting in an explosive rage is prompted by a fundamental need to control. It is that need, however unconscious, which triggers off the violence.

Finally, the fact that many men effectively abuse their partners emotionally and psychologically, without using anger or physical violence at all, surely shows just how much they are in control of the situation.

### 'It is all a matter of low self-esteem'

Many abusers have low self-esteem. They do not feel good about themselves. They wish they were different. And because they feel so insecure they often adopt another 'image'. Their fears and emotions are masked by controlling, abusive behaviour. They will mock their partners, put them down and lash out at them with fists and words. They convince themselves of their own importance and feel justified in keeping their women in check.

In reality, however, these men are dependent on their partners for this sense of power and superiority. They feel inadequate and worthless, but they cannot admit it. Often, too, they are frightened of real intimacy. The only relationships they can have are ones in which they feel they call all the shots.

However, the issue of men's low self-esteem is only a factor in woman abuse, not the root cause. This is underlined by the fact that many men have low self-esteem, but do not abuse their partners, and although both men and women experience feelings of worthlessness and insecurity, only a tiny proportion of women abuse men. When a woman feels insecure and dependent, she does not behave in the same way. Also, there are many men who have low self-esteem, but never abuse their wives and girlfriends – so there must be some other cause.

Many people also argue that only women who have low self-esteem can be abused, but I dispute this. It is true that abusers often seek out women who are lacking in self-esteem, because they are easier to dominate. It is also true that women have inherited a tradition which brands them inferior to men. They live in a society in which their self-esteem is not fostered. I would argue that for most abused women low self-esteem is a *consequence* of the abuse, not a cause. Many women start out in a relationship with high self-esteem, which is systematically broken when the men they fall in love with humiliate, hit and undermine them. However confident and comfortable with themselves they may once have been, they now begin to believe it when their abusers tell them that they are bad or crazy or that it is their fault that the men behave the way they do.

The danger of this particular myth is that once again it focuses the problem on the women. But the problem does not lie with the women – whether they have high self-esteem or low self-esteem. It lies with men and the society in which they live. We have to ask the question: will boosting a woman's self-esteem stop her partner from being violent? The answer is no. A woman cannot make a man abusive. It is always his choice.

I am not disputing that drink, stress, jealousy, low self-esteem and other such problems can play a part in woman abuse – but I do not accept that they are the cause. Solving any or all of these problems will not end the abuse of women. And concentrating on them only diverts attention from the real issue, excuses the abusers and perpetuates the abuse. Because, for as long as it is convenient to be distracted by myths, no one feels the need to do anything about it.

I believe that the cause of woman abuse is more fundamental. Only by looking at our society and culture as a whole can we answer the question: why do men abuse women?

# CHAPTER 5

# Why Men Abuse Women

## Men are more important

The way you see a problem determines what you do about it, so if you see woman abuse as being caused by a man drinking too much, you simply send him to Alcoholics Anonymous. If you think it is about a woman's masochism, you send her to an analyst to delve into her subconscious. If you think a man is suffering from some chemical deficiency, you simply administer the appropriate drugs. Many of these factors, which I discussed in the previous chapter, do contribute to abuse, but they do not *cause* it. Woman abuse is the culmination of certain factors.

Deborah Sinclair suggested, in her book *Understanding Wife Assault*,[52] that three major elements interlock to perpetuate the problem: first, the psychological experiences of the individual men and women (jealousy, fear of abandonment, low self-esteem, stress); second, the lack of resources (housing, lack of childcare); and third, the negative responses of the community to the problem (the failure to prosecute, and the attitude of a society which asks 'What did you do to make him hit you?' and 'It takes two...').

Chapters 3 and 4 have looked at these factors. In this chapter I am going to focus on the third major factor: society's beliefs about and attitudes towards the roles of men and women. This is the root cause of woman abuse – and it is also what allows woman abuse, in all its forms, to continue.

The harrowing statistics on violence against women will not change unless we admit that woman abuse is a symptom of our unequal society. Many policy-makers find this talk of gender uncomfortable and old-fashioned. They would rather see it as a crime just like any other – a problem, yes, but not one that requires serious introspection about the way we all live our lives. Of course, sweeping misogyny under the rug is the easier option – then all we need to do is to root out the 'bad eggs'.

This will achieve little, though. Until we challenge the social norms that have led men to believe they are allowed to abuse women, the violence will not be reduced. That is why I am choosing to highlight some of the myriad ways women are marginalised and silenced in our society, so that we might begin to challenge them.

For a long time, Sally was unable to see that Guy's behaviour had nothing to do with *her*, that she did not cause his behaviour, that nothing she tried would change it. Finally, she was able to accept that she was in no way to blame. Nor could she excuse his behaviour with any of society's myths. It was not because he had occasionally drunk too much, because he was under stress at work, or because he was a jealous person. She began to see that what had really been happening was that Guy had been controlling her in a host of subtle ways. And that the responsibility for what he was doing was his. He had learned to behave that way long before he ever met Sally.

Without any prompting, when she came to see me she would tell me that she had noticed similar behaviour in men all around her. 'My best friend's husband does exactly the same thing,' she would say. 'He's always putting her down.' Or 'I can't believe the way my sister has stopped seeing her friends because her boyfriend wants her to be with him all the time.'

'Why are men like that?' she asked. Women who have come to recognise the controlling patterns of their partner's behaviour ask that question all the time. 'I suppose I always thought in terms of men being somehow in charge, but I never thought it was relevant to what was happening to me,' says Rebecca.

I suggested to Sally and Rebecca that the answer to the question 'Why are men like that?' is that they are simply doing on an individual level what men do on a larger scale. The way Guy and Ralph had treated them was just a reflection of the way men treat women in society as a whole. When Guy was grudging about allowing Sally money, he was echoing a society which allows women to earn only 80 per cent of the amount that men earn,[53] in spite of equal-pay legislation. When Ralph isolated Rebecca from her friends by turning down invitations and trying to stop her from working, he was behaving the way men behave to women on a much bigger scale, by expecting them to stay at home with their children, forcing them to curtail their social activities and trapping them inside their houses.

When James humiliated and degraded Laura by putting her down in front of their friends and subjecting her to the kind of sexual abuse which made her feel ashamed and unclean, he was just doing what men do on a larger scale: putting them down through the kind of advertising which uses women as 'objects' to sell cars or cocktails, and degrading them through pornography and rape.

'So what?' you might say. 'What has men using women's bodies to sell cars got to do with woman abuse?' People are always telling me: 'That is just feminist gobbledygook.' But it is not just gobbledygook. There really is a very strong link between the way men treat women in society and the way they abuse them in the home. If men do not respect women on a universal level, there will always be some men who will treat their wives and girlfriends with the same contempt.

Okay, so women like Emmeline Pankhurst no longer have to chain themselves to railings; but if it is really true that men and women are equal, how come many men walk away scot-free when they bruise and batter their wives? And, more to the point, on any given day why is Refuge supporting thousands of women and children who have suffered horrifying emotional and physical scars at the hands of men? Why is it that so many women are afraid to be themselves, to have their own friends, to express their opinions? Why do they spend their lives avoiding anything which might upset their partners, for fear of retribution?

Frankly, the reality is that men and women are still not equal. Men are still seen to be superior, and women are still discriminated against. The bottom line is that men have the power and the control, and women are denied it. When one sex is given all the power and control, it is inevitable that there will be some men who will abuse it, and feel entitled to keep their wives and girlfriends in line, even if that means using abusive behaviour to get their own way.

What I hope to show in this chapter is that, however far we think we have come, very little has changed since St Paul wrote in a letter to the Corinthians that the man 'is the image and glory of God, but the woman is the glory of the man'. In too many cases, woman abuse is only a short step away.

Nowhere is the idea that men are the dominant sex more clearly expressed than in the institution of marriage. 'Who giveth this woman?' the priest asks in the traditional Church of England wedding service, before going on to demand that she 'love, honour and obey' her husband. For centuries, marriage has given men a 'free pass' to abuse 'his woman' – rape in marriage only became illegal in 1991 and it is still legal for a man to rape his wife in 38 countries around the world.[54]

Since I wrote the first edition of this book, the number of women getting married has reduced. Today, 90 per cent of 60-year-olds have married, whereas it is estimated that only 50 per cent of today's young adults will do so.[55] And yet women and girls continue to be bombarded with images of marriage as the ultimate marker of success.

Tips on catching and keeping a man still dominate magazine front pages. Glossy photo-features lauding celebrities who have managed to achieve the 'perfect' family jostle for space alongside screaming headlines about women who 'just can't hold on to a man'. One only has to think of model and actress Jerry Hall's famous quote, 'My mother said it was simple to keep a man: you must be a maid in the living room, a cook in the kitchen and a whore in the bedroom. I said I'd hire the other two and take care of the bedroom bit', to get the picture.

Just like when I wrote the first edition, the biggest media event of the decade involved a huge white dress and a princess –

this time William and Kate rather than Charles and Diana. Still, marriage is depicted as the 'happy ever after' fairy tale. Every inch of Kate's wedding day was pored over and promoted in minute detail by the media. It was the most important international news story for days. Even if fewer women are marrying in practice, it is clear that this orange-blossom ideal – that marriage will bring ultimate happiness and everything else is unimportant – is alive and well. Once you have a ring on your finger, that's it: happy ever after.

Melinda, like many of the women I meet, had been brought up on these ideals. 'I suppose I was looking for the special kind of love my mother and father shared. They really are made for each other,' she explained. 'It's a marriage made in heaven. I had a career, and I had my own home, but I always thought that if I got married, then I'd have what they had. And I thought it would be a "happy ever after" type of thing.'

However, far from the hearts and flowers ideal, the reality of marriage for women frequently turns out to be something entirely different. Charlotte Fedders (see Chapter 1) could not believe her luck when she met and married her lawyer husband John. She did not really believe that she deserved such a wonderful man. Fedders, on the other hand, saw in Charlotte someone who would bow down to his every wish, without questioning, someone who accepted that she was in no way his equal.

To love, honour and obey – the words sound noble and romantic but, for many women whose men hold such beliefs, abuse is only a step away. 'I think I became James's property after we got married,' says Laura, looking back. 'I don't think I was before. And I hadn't reckoned on that, because that's not how I think about things at all.' Hazel says, 'The day Jimmy and I got married, he said to me, "You are my property now", and that made me uneasy. Just for a moment, I thought, "God, what have I done? I am *his*."' The brief niggle vanished, because she was convinced she was going to live happily ever after.

And, as we have seen, it is not only married women who are in danger. Charm Syndrome Man is looking for commitment, but there need not be a wedding ring involved. Sally says, 'Guy and I weren't married, but we might as well have been. All that was missing was the piece of paper. If we had got married, I doubt if I would have promised to love, honour and obey – but it wouldn't have made any difference to his attitude. I think that's the way he expected me to behave, anyway.'

'But men and women are equal these days,' people say. 'The women in my office earn just as much as me,' men insist. 'My wife and I have a perfectly equal relationship. We take all the decisions together,' they say. 'I have a woman boss,' they argue. But does that woman boss have a husband who is at home ironing her clothes, cooking her evening meal and looking after the children, or does she come home from work and do it herself?

Perhaps her husband does do as much around the house as she does. But such a couple – where household chores and childcare are split 50/50 and the woman reaches her full potential – must push against huge barriers in order to achieve equality.

Take parental leave. When women have a baby, they are entitled to 39 weeks of statutory maternity pay – often topped up by their employer. For men, paternity leave is two weeks – and less than 10 per cent of men take more.[56] This is just one way in which women are pushed into the role of primary caregiver. Of course, many women want to take on this role – but the point is, they should have a choice.

The Government's 'Shared Parental Leave' scheme, introduced in April 2015, whereby both parents can share up to 50 weeks of leave, 39 with some pay, was lauded as a huge step forward – but since the scheme was introduced, only a tiny number of men have opted for shared leave, and one survey found that 80 per cent of employees said a decision to do so would depend on finances.[57] There is a semblance of choice – but only for those who can afford it.

If a couple decides that one parent should care for the child – perhaps because childcare is prohibitively expensive – then who is it likely to be? Thanks to a stubborn gender pay gap of almost 20 per cent,[58] many couples simply cannot afford for the mother to continue with her career.

Employers are still reluctant to give women jobs which involve long-term planning and commitment, because they expect them to abandon their work to have children. I hear stories all the time of women not being offered contracts or partnerships for this very reason, however insistent the women are that they are single-minded about their jobs and have no intention of having children at that time. Forty-one per cent of women work part-time, compared to 12 per cent of men[59] – and part-time workers earn less. Again, women are left with less money and less power, a fact that some men – consciously or unconsciously – choose to abuse.

By giving men the dominant role, the institution of marriage still denies women real choices. But even in the most forward-thinking of relationships, again and again, women sacrifice their careers to raise children because society makes it almost impossible to do anything else. In doing so, women often become financially dependent on their partners, and isolated from the outside interests, stimulation and relationships which working in a job can bring. They often deny their own talents by supporting their husbands while they go through further education. Many women tell me that they have taken menial jobs in order to pay for their husbands to go to law school or medical school. Often in these cases the men walk out on them; the women are left with boring jobs and no money while the men start new lives on a high income, thanks to the women's sacrifices.

Ninety per cent of single-parent families are headed by women. These households are nearly twice as likely to be in poverty as couple-parent families. Almost half of separated mothers do not receive any payment from estranged fathers towards their children.[60] When fathers do pay up, it is often a measly amount: the average was £41 a week at the time of writing.[61] Men, who may very well have forced their wives to be dependent on them financially, get away with abandoning their responsibilities.

'Charm Syndrome' is a term I have invented, but the behaviour it describes is as old as civilisation. Historically, women have always been regarded as chattels to be handed over in marriage. 'But we have come a long way since the days when men "owned" their women like goods and chattels,' I hear you say. But have we? When Pamela, the eponymous heroine of Samuel Richardson's eighteenth-century novel, speaks about 'Mr. B's rules for marriage', I hear Rebecca talking about Ralph, or Melinda talking about Trevor. The language is different, but the sentiments are remarkably similar.

Says Pamela:
> *I must think his displeasure the heaviest thing that can befall me [...] And so, that I must not wish to incur it, to save my body else from it [...] I must bear with him, even when I find him in the wrong [...] He insists upon it, that a woman should give her husband reason to think she prefers him before all men.*

Says Mr. B:
> *If she overcomes, it must be by sweetness and compliance [...] She must not shew reluctance, uneasiness or doubt, to oblige him; and that too at half a word, and must not be bidden twice to do one thing. In all companies a wife must shew respect and love to her husband.*[62]

Even when women have jobs outside the home, they still do the lion's share of the housework, catering to their partner's specific needs at the expense of their own. They are expected to be Superwomen, juggling job and home. At the same time they must never neglect their partner's emotional needs. Frequently such women find themselves exhausted from doing half a dozen jobs, while the men only have to concentrate on one. In 2014, parenting website Mumsnet asked almost 1,000 working mothers about who does what in the home. Seventy-one per cent of women are responsible for the weekly clean, 77 per cent are responsible for washing, and 70 per cent are responsible for cooking for the kids.[63]

Society teaches women that their role is to look after home and family, to be the emotional ballast; the fact that she works full time or has other independent commitments does not give her a free pass. Even if the chores are divided more evenly, invariably the 'emotional labour' falls on her shoulders. Her husband might be willing to do the cooking and cleaning, but who does the school call first if there is ever a problem? According to Mumsnet, it is the mothers 80 per cent of the time. The same applies for all manner of responsibilities that could broadly be described as 'caring' – 77 per cent of working mums are responsible for buying birthday gifts; 88 per cent manage doctors' appointments. Working women have all the responsibility, stresses and strains of their day jobs. But they also have their 'second job', this time unpaid – that of carer and comforter, cook and cleaner, personal assistant and chauffeur.

Men, on the other hand, are still perceived as the breadwinners, the key decision-makers, the heads of the family. 'Wait till your father gets home' is the threat that many children grow up with and never shake off. Rebecca laughingly admits that she used to bounce on the sofa with the children while Ralph was away – because he forbade her to even sit on it.

We are steeped in the tradition of men being the dominant sex. Men are given the power and control which can be so dangerous. Even when women reject that tradition, they often find themselves trapped by it nonetheless, thanks to deeply entrenched patriarchal attitudes. So when people ask 'Why do men abuse women?', one answer is simply 'Because they always have done'.

Charm Syndrome Man sees his partner as the rightful object of his authority. He believes he can control her actions, even her thoughts. And even when his behaviour becomes intolerable, she is trapped into staying in the relationship because society says she must. 'For the sake of the children,' people say, or 'It's up to you to make it work.'

No matter how equal women appear to others or how many crucial decisions they make at work every day, many women are so conditioned into believing that their happiness is tied up with pleasing their partner and creating the 'perfect' home that they are often unable to reject this notion. If they do so, they risk being branded 'ranting feminists'.

The result of such conditioning is that it widens even further the gulf between men and women in terms of power. He goes on thinking he is superior and has the power to treat his partner in any way he thinks is right, while she believes it is her responsibility to make things work. In such an unequal partnership it is inevitable that some men are always going to resort to violence and abuse to enforce their sense of superiority.

## So men call all the shots

As I have pointed out, men abuse women because they are allowed to do so – and have always been allowed to do so. For as long as men have considered that a woman's life revolves around her man, that her role is to love, honour and obey him – for better or for worse – there have been secular laws and moral codes which have given men the go-ahead to underline that idea with abuse. And even in this so-called enlightened age, when such barbaric laws have been abolished (at least in this country), the thinking behind them still prevails.

The history books are peppered with codes and laws which enforce the idea that if women do not behave as men think they should, they can be punished. As long ago as 2500 BC, if a woman argued with her husband, her name was engraved on a brick which was then used to smash out her teeth.

In the fifteenth century, one Friar Cherubino of Siena produced a volume called *The Rules of Marriage*. He instructed:

> *When you see your wife commit an offence, don't rush at her with insults and violent blows; rather, first correct the wrong lovingly and pleasantly, and sweetly teach her not to do it again so as not to offend God, injure her soul, or bring shame upon herself or you...*

However, if that does not work, he advises: 'Scold her sharply, bully and terrify her.' And if *that* is not enough, 'Take a stick and beat her soundly... not in rage, but out of charity and concern for her soul, so that the beating will rebound to your merit and her good.'[64]

The Koran gives a similar message: 'Men are the managers of the affairs of women. Righteous women are therefore obedient and those you fear may be rebellious admonish. Banish them to their couches and beat them.'

The idea that men were entitled to chastise their wives was echoed in secular law. Even in the relatively civilised era of Charles I, it was accepted that a man could beat his wife – but not after dark, as that might disturb the peace.

Most people have heard the phrase 'rule of thumb', but not so many know that it refers to the common law tradition that allowed a man to chastise his wife, so long as it was with a stick no thicker than his thumb – and that is about the size of a broomstick!

Things seemed to be looking up in 1861, when the Offences Against the Person Act made assault a crime. Surely now women would be safe? Not so. Only eight years later the philosopher John Stuart Mill wrote:

> *From the very earliest twilight of human society, every woman [...] was found in a state of bondage to some man. [...]*
>
> *How vast is the number of men, in any great country, who are little higher than brutes, and [...] this never prevents them from being able, through the laws of marriage, to obtain a victim [...]*
>
> *The vilest malefactor has some wretched woman tied to him, against whom he can commit any atrocity except killing her and, if tolerably cautious, can do that without much danger of legal penalty.*[65]

And in 1878 Frances Power Cobbe published a report called *Wife Torture in England*. She asked, 'What reasons can be alleged... why the male of the human species should be the only animal which maltreats its mate, or any female of its own kind?'[66]

That is a very good question – to which the only answer can be that man is the only animal brought up in a society which encourages him to behave in such a way, and then turns a blind eye. Today, men still assault women because rarely does anyone stop them from doing so. Even though the law in theory offers protection, in practice it fails to provide it, again and again. As I have already written, all too often the police still do not arrest and charge offenders, and Crown Prosecutors fail to prosecute.

Our society has not really changed so much since the twelfth century, when the monk Gratian decreed that it is a natural human order that women should serve their husbands.[67]

As Hazel's parish priest advised her whenever she turned to him for help: 'Marriage is a sacred thing. I know it can be difficult at times, but it is your duty to love your husband and look after him.'

Another cleric advised a woman who had been attacked by her husband with a hammer and chisel to do the same thing. He told her he would make her husband swear on the Bible never to do it again, and then she should go home to him. Six months later she turned up at a refuge with further injuries.

When I asked Sally about her background and her life before she met Guy, she told me: 'I had always been brought up with the idea that I was nothing without a man, that having a career was all well and good, but not at the expense of a husband and family.' The more I asked women the same question, the more I became convinced that no matter how high-powered their jobs, no matter how intelligent or well-off the women were, they were all brought up to think that their ultimate happiness depended on a man.

Hazel says, 'I think what I was looking for subconsciously when I met Jimmy was a man, a husband, to protect me and be a father to my children. I didn't want much – I didn't want to be rich, to have power, or to be famous. I didn't want a fancy car, or a lot of material possessions. I really didn't expect much. I just wanted a man, a house and two kids. That was what I was looking for. And Jimmy was lovely, he was gorgeous. There I was thinking, "I've got what I wanted." Of course it wasn't to be...'

Finding a man who has a good job, is reliable and makes a nice income is also seen to be a kind of status symbol. Telling the story of Charlotte Fedders and her husband John in *Shattered Dreams*, Laura Elliott writes: 'On the outside John was the knight that she and her affluent, Catholic school girlfriends had been taught to want – the handsome, ambitious breadwinner, through whom they could vicariously be successes.'[68] Charlotte's upbringing had led her to place an enormous emphasis on this idea of achieving status through a man who could support her.

Both men and women search for that certain someone and that certain chemistry which sets pulses racing, making them feel special, important, fulfilled. Both men and women sing love songs and write love poetry. Yet for women there is this extra emphasis – imbued through popular culture and reinforced by sexism which stacks the odds against women – that without a man they are nothing.

Women are brought up with this warning ringing in their ears: 'You don't want to be left on the shelf, dear.' What a cruel expression, with its connotation of goods no one wants. In just the same way, the word 'spinster' acquired connotations of someone old and wizened and prim, with no experience of men – but call an unmarried man a 'bachelor' and the automatic image is of someone handsome, eligible, a 'bit of a rogue' with women.

Despite shouts of 'Men and women are equal these days!' society still encourages women to be dependent, to believe that they are unable to stand on their own feet, and that they have to rely on men for protection, stability and support. Women who are dependent have less power, and they feel less able to challenge the norm. They do not believe they have rights. Nor do men – who have, of course, absorbed the same message. When men fall in love it tends to be only a part of their life, rather than an all-consuming thing. Their careers are equally, often more, important. As Lord Byron wrote in *Don Juan*:

> Man's love is of man's life a thing apart,
> 'Tis woman's whole existence.[69]

The result is a dangerous inequality between the sexes. As long as women are trapped in this way, some men will always exploit them.

As I explained to Sally and Rebecca, the controlling behaviour they suffered at the hands of Guy and Ralph were only symptoms of a much wider problem. The way abusive men behave towards their partners is magnified on a much larger scale in society as a whole. And women are no more responsible for that than they are in their individual relationships.

When people insist that men and women are equal these days, I say, 'Look around you.' It simply is not true. Certainly we have had two female prime ministers, there is a Sex Discrimination Act and we do see some women pilots, engineers and road sweepers. There are more women in Parliament than ever before. Women in public life are now permitted to exist – that much, at least, is progress – but they still face huge barriers. Long hours, archaic traditions and the need to split time between Westminster and a local constituency mean many women find being an MP incompatible with family life. Not so for men. A 2012 survey found that almost half of women MPs have no children, compared to just 28 per cent of male MPs. Women who have children are more likely to enter Parliament when their children are older than the children of male MPs.[70]

Yet women MPs are often penalised for not having children. 'What is wrong with them that they haven't been able to keep a man and procreate?' the public asks. 'Are they just selfish?' Rosie Campbell, one of the academics who conducted the research cited above sums it up: 'For men, having a wife and children is a political resource, whereas for women, not having children was the thing that gave them the time to do politics.'[71]

The same is true in other professions. The UK has one of the lowest proportions of female judges in Europe, at just 25 per cent in 2016.[72] As you can see, women – and particularly mothers – are locked out of careers in which they could improve the lot of other women. In schools, we often tell girls that they can be anything they want to be – the sky is the limit. Girls consistently outperform boys at school, and women are now 35 per cent more likely than men to go to university[73] – and yet we still see far fewer women in top jobs. Many of those young women are in for a rude awakening when they enter the workplace or begin thinking about having children. Motherhood is wonderful but it is also a trap – because society makes it so.

If a woman decides to stay at home and enjoys bringing up her children, it should be because that is what she wants to do. She should not feel pushed into a role which is expected of her. Nor should men feel trapped in the role of breadwinner. They should be free to hand that role over to their partner if that is what makes them both happy. Yet the truth is that men's jobs are always given more status; even single fathers get more praise and attention than single mothers. Men and women have been saturated with these ideas for so long that, however enlightened we may think we are, we are still locked into the idea that men are entitled to be in charge.

Women who do reach positions of power and put their head above the parapet also face huge hostility, particularly when they talk about 'women's issues'. Aside from mainstream media headlines that fixate on their looks, or their relationships, or the fact that they should just 'give us a smile', women in public life also face a barrage of abuse online. As men see women acquire power, many feel the need to put them in their place and limit their voice. The think tank DEMOS studied the extent of misogynistic abuse online in 2016. It monitored the use of the words 'slut' and 'whore' by Twitter users, and found that in just three weeks, 6,500 individuals were targeted by 10,000 misogynistic tweets.

Often abuse online is dismissed as 'not as serious'. Women are told simply to get off Twitter or Facebook and to just ignore it. But the psychological impact of a man publishing a woman's home address online, inciting others to abuse her, or threatening to kill and rape her, should not be underestimated. The feminist activist Caroline Criado-Perez is a case in point. Having campaigned for Jane Austen to be depicted on the new £10 bank note, in 2013 she was subjected to a barrage of Twitter abuse and threats of rape. Similarly, the classicist and TV academic Professor Mary Beard regularly received online misogynistic tweets because she refused to wear make-up and was even tweeted a bomb threat. Speaking about her experience to the *Guardian*, Caroline Criado-Perez described how the abuse made her feel: 'I felt really sick, to be honest. And horrified. It's not like I didn't know this happened to women, but to see it in front of you, directed at you [...] I've got this fear and tension bubbling up underneath the surface all the time. And I guess that's why really I can't eat.' On the subject of social media and misogyny, she says: 'It's been going on for millennia.

Women have always been put in their place and kept there through the threat of sexual violence.'[74]

It is not just high-profile women who experience abuse of this kind. The women using Refuge's services frequently tell us that their perpetrators have abused them on social media, including verbal abuse and harassment, and trying to humiliate them via social media. One woman's perpetrator doctored photographs of her to make it look like she was with other men, and shared them with her family and friends. Another abuser took over his wife's Facebook and used it to have sexually explicit conversations with women. Online abuse should not be seen in a vacuum; misogyny on social media fuels contempt for women. Through her pioneering 'Everyday Sexism' project[75] – a blog that documents the daily bouts of sexism women and girls experience – Laura Bates was able to demonstrate the way in which sexism touches every aspect of women's lives. From being groped on public transport, to being catcalled on the street, to being talked over in a meeting – the blog shows the myriad ways in which men dominate and demean women. Even without a 'serious' incident of abuse, women, whether members of the Cabinet or teenagers in college, may be cowed, curtailed – and ultimately controlled – by a thousand cuts. Seeing women in positions of power is one thing – but we will not see real progress until all women are permitted to reach their full potential, unencumbered by male abuse.

Online abuse may be a new method of control, but discrimination is age-old. Women are barely less discriminated against than they were between the fifteenth and eighteenth centuries when some nine million women in Europe and America were stigmatised as witches and burned at the stake because they challenged men's authority by running their estates and businesses when their husbands were at war or had died of plague. Other women who challenged the monopoly of male physicians by using country remedies for healing met the same fate.

Have we really made such great strides since the days when women were denied the vote, when they had to adopt male pseudonyms to write their novels because otherwise they laid themselves open to accusations of neglecting their husbands and families? Are we really any more inclined to see the world as a place where women are important than we did when our only view of history was coloured by men and their attitudes and beliefs, male explorers, male scientists, male composers, male writers giving us *their* view of the world? Where are the women? Names like Elizabeth Browning and Jane Austen are exceptions; they are not the rule.

Women may be referred to as 'the power behind the throne' but that expression makes them even more invisible. Many women have had to fulfil their own ambitions through their sons or their husbands because they have not been allowed to do so themselves. The woman's role is to nurture her men towards power and success. The man is the one who gets all the credit and all the glory.

In all sorts of subtle ways, all these historical references are more stitches in the tapestry of woman abuse. Men believe they have the right to control and dominate women because they have historically been given that right. We are saturated – all of us – with the idea that men call the shots. Given this, it is understandable that women sometimes internalise these patriarchal attitudes. Women say to me all the time 'I prefer the company of men to women', or 'I'd rather work with men than women' – what they are really saying is that men, to them, are more important, so they want to be associated with them rather than with women, whom they see (probably unconsciously) as inferior. Just as individual women tend to deny what is happening to them – because facing up to it means taking difficult and often painful decisions – women as a whole do the same thing. It is easier to deny reality by accepting the traditional notion that men are supposed to be in charge. The idea is so ingrained in us all that we do not even notice it half the time. However, it is there and, as long as it remains, so does the problem of woman abuse.

## And women get the bit parts

From an early age women are taught that men are important and women get the bit parts. In traditional children's books it is Mother Bear who wears the pinny and makes the cakes, while Father Bear goes out to work. Mothers in these children's stories rarely do or say anything challenging. They are never seen making important decisions. They simply make the sandwiches for picnics, cook the supper and wash the clothes.

Publishers may be more aware of gender stereotyping now, but children's books are still regularly labelled with 'for boys' or 'for girls'. An American study published in 2011 found a huge gender disparity, with male central characters far outnumbering female characters. According to the researchers:

> The messages conveyed through representation of males and females in books contribute to children's ideas of what it means to be a boy, girl, man, or woman. The disparities we find point to the symbolic annihilation of women and girls, and particularly female animals, in 20th-century children's literature, suggesting to children that these characters are less important than their male counterparts… The disproportionate numbers of males in central roles may encourage children to accept the invisibility of women and girls and to believe they are less important than men and boys, thereby reinforcing the gender system.[76]

Despite a vogue for adverts and magazines aimed at the career woman, the advertiser's favourite image of a woman is still either the temptress draped over a sleek, sexy new car, the housewife fretting over how she can get little Johnny's sports shirt clean for the morning, or how many plates she can wash up with a particular brand of liquid. Men, on the other hand, discuss the finer points of an important business deal while they jet across the Atlantic, or wax lyrical about their favourite pint of bitter in the pub, leaving their wives at home. The result of such stereotyping is that neither men nor women have real choices about their roles.

Another way in which men are able to maintain control over women is by devaluing them in all kinds of ways: on television, in pornography and through prostitution, in advertising which uses women in sexy attire to sell sports cars, and in newspapers and magazines. Whenever a woman is draped naked over the centrefold of a men's magazine, the message is that women are there simply to titillate men. If women are cheapened and treated as objects, is it any wonder that in their individual relationships men feel entitled to treat them badly?

Pornography is not sexy or erotic. Pornography is about degrading women and portraying them as servile, sexual objects, with a status which is little higher than that of an animal. Often such 'titillation' is linked with violence: women are shown in bondage or being mutilated. A 2010 US study found that 88 per cent of the pornography scenes they studied contained physical aggression, principally gagging, spanking and slapping.[77] Almost half the scenes included verbal aggression – primarily name-calling. Women are dehumanised – and these images are now served up to younger and younger boys, on internet browsers and mobile phones. Is it any wonder that many young men do not understand the need for consent in sex? It is a horrifying fact that 30 per cent of rape victims are girls under 16 years of age.[78]

Pornography, rape and sexual harassment serve as reminders of the threat that always hangs over women. While stalking is considered to be a criminal offence and is recognised as a direct form of harassment, women's lives continue to be governed by fear. Because women are unable to walk the streets freely, because they are told they should not wear 'provocative' clothing, or say things which could be construed as encouraging men to 'take advantage' of them, they are isolated, their social lives are curtailed, they are denied the same freedom that men have. Ironically, women are taught that they need male protection against these very things. Rape is more than a violent crime – it underlines the lack of respect with which men treat women. One of the earliest laws on rape is to be found in the Book of Deuteronomy:

> *If a man find a damsel that is a virgin, that is not*
> *betrothed, and lay hold on her, and lie with her, and they*
> *be found: then the man that lay with her shall give unto*
> *the damsel's father fifty shekels of silver, and she shall be*
> *his wife…*

In other words, the father gets compensation for damaged goods and the daughter's 'compensation' is marriage to the rapist.

'But that was a long time ago,' people will say. So it was, but the attitudes it illustrates have changed very little. After all, men do not always receive stiff punishment for rape. Approximately 85,000 women are raped every year in England and Wales. Yet only 5.7 per cent of reported rape cases end in a conviction.[79] Even nowadays, a woman's sexual history can be brought up in court, as in the recent case of Ched Evans – a professional footballer accused of raping a 19-year-old woman. After being convicted of rape in 2012, Evans appealed the verdict. This time, at the retrial, jurors were permitted to hear from two witnesses who gave testimony about the woman's sexual preferences and the language she used during sex, thanks to a loophole in the legislation which usually bans this practice. Evans was acquitted. Despite the fact that using this kind of evidence is supposed to be an exception, the case potentially sets a dangerous precedent – and it showed the extent to which juries, made up of ordinary members of the public, in some cases may be ready to believe a woman was 'asking for it'. It is a measure of how little attention society pays to the rights of women and how women frequently have to convince a court that they were not to blame for an attack. Still, it will be suggested that the woman provoked the attack by walking alone late at night or wearing short skirts. This victim-blaming attitude is unsurprising – even police forces display posters which tell women what they should and shouldn't do in order to avoid sexual assault. In 2015, one force circulated a poster which read: 'Which one of your mates is most vulnerable on a night out? The one you leave behind. Many sexual assaults could be prevented. Stick together and don't let your friend leave with a stranger or go off on their own.' It tells women to alter their behaviour in order to avoid rape – rather than telling men not to rape. Following widespread criticism, the force scrapped the poster and issued an apology.[80]

Posters like this are not just one-off blunders; they are symptomatic of a society that fails to recognise that rape, like assault by men on their partners, is a calculated act of violence and has nothing to do with uncontrollable sexual urges. At some point the rapist makes a choice and, whatever the woman's behaviour, she cannot force a man to rape or assault her. A 2017 Fawcett Society study exposed how many men fail to grasp this. In answer to the question 'If a woman goes out late at night, wearing a short skirt, gets drunk and is then the victim of a sexual assault, is she totally or partly to blame?', 41 per cent of men aged 18–24 said she was.[81]

From the cradle almost, men and women are brought up to see their roles in life as different: he is dominant, she is dependent. There is no escaping the fact that little girls are brought up differently from little boys.

Boys frequently grow up sneering at displays of emotion or at gentle pastimes, for fear of being considered 'soft' or 'sissies'. They are brought up to be tough, to play with guns and tanks and dumper trucks, and show their aggression on the football pitch and the rugby field. They are taught that boys should take control, be forceful, be dominant. Aggressive play is too often considered healthy in a little boy.

Girls, on the other hand, are encouraged to be sweet, affectionate and compliant. They are taught that girls should be self-sacrificing and caring. They are dressed up like little dolls in frothy outfits which stop them from expressing themselves in the rough and tumble world of their brothers, and they are given dolls' houses and ironing boards and toy vacuum cleaners.

As Linda Tschirhart Sanford and Mary Ellen Donovan note in *Women and Self-Esteem*, 'Boys are encouraged to fight back when others try to violate them, and as a result many males unfortunately see violence as the normal way to try to resolve a variety of problems. Girls, however, are encouraged to do nothing, and the helplessness a girl learned in childhood often carries over into adulthood, where passivity seems the only way to handle problems . . .' Little girls who grow up absorbing such attitudes expect few choices to be available to them. They expect to be 'given away' in marriage, and to become the property of their husbands. Little boys grow up expecting their partners to be subordinate to them.

The idea that men are the important, dominant sex, on whom women depend for their happiness, is reinforced in the story books which play such an important part in forming children's attitudes. Little girls grow up with the image of the Lady in all those knight-in-shining-armour epics, or the Sleeping Beauty, the beautiful maiden who can only be brought to life by her handsome prince. Instead of helping herself, Sleeping Beauty has to wait passively to be rescued. The myth – set up by the male writers of such books and supported by a society which has been advocating such ideas for centuries – is that women are helpless, passive, servile creatures who cannot think for themselves, while the men have the important, active roles. Consequently women grow up with the idea that they do not have power and control over their own lives. And men grow up with the idea that women are powerless creatures simply waiting to be turned on by them.

The knight in shining armour was the champion of God crusading through Europe, waging war on infidels and (in the tradition of courtly love) wooing beautiful, submissive and untouchable women from afar. But since the whole ethos of courtly love depended on the fact that the knight conducted his courtship of his lady by remote control, there was no question of any kind of real relationship. The woman was simply a symbol, an object through which the knight could show off his valour and gallantry.

For the woman's part, the knight in shining armour became the romantic ideal: but what did he really represent? A charming but domineering character who took all the initiatives and believed in using violence to enforce his beliefs. Where have we heard that before?

When the little girl grows up, she receives the same messages from popular songs and novels. In a hit London musical, the heroine sings dreamily of the power her hero has to move her, to change, mould and *improve* her. The words suggest that both the heroine and hero assume that *he* has the right to fashion *her* in any way he pleases. Boys too are susceptible to the message in such lyrics.

A similar idea is perpetuated in the Mills and Boon-style romantic novel. It is true that a whole new wave of best-selling novels, soap operas and TV mini-series has spawned a different kind of heroine: the independent, glamorous woman who claws her way to the top of a business empire by her perfectly manicured fingernails, giving every male in sight hell on the way. But it is the novelty of the idea which gives it such instant appeal. And such dramas invariably conclude with the woman realising that her work is meaningless without the love of a good man – invariably a hero tough enough and powerful enough not to take no for an answer, even from her. In rejecting the weak characters she meets along the way, in favour of the strong man who takes control, this kind of heroine is still reinforcing the traditional idea that men should take the dominant role. If a woman is strong and capable, it simply requires an even stronger, even more powerful man to take her in hand.

Throughout our culture the idea that a woman might have potential is pushed to one side. The lesson is: men should be looking for women who will fulfil all their needs, while they go out into the big wide world and develop their potential: women should be searching for the Prince Charming who will sweep her off to live happily ever after.

I believe that having sowed the seeds of woman abuse, society (albeit tacitly) gives men permission to go on controlling and abusing their partners – by turning a blind eye to the abuse, blaming the women, perpetuating the myths about the causes of abuse and failing to provide adequate care, facilities and, above all, legal protection for women who have suffered at the hands of abusive men.

Of course, not all men who grow up receiving such signals from society go on to abuse women. When all the analysis is done, the truth is that men *always have a choice*. It may be very difficult for them to shake off the messages they have been bombarded with since they were children, but they still have the choice whether or not to abuse women. They can turn away, and take a different course. It is up to society to make them do that. But society cannot do that until it stops shirking the issue and accepts that gender inequality is the real cause of woman abuse. Once we can all accept that, we can try to work together to find a way forward.

# CHAPTER 6

# The Way Forward

## For women

'For so long,' says Melinda, 'I carried on rather than face the horror. I couldn't think of myself as abused, because it was just too unacceptable. I couldn't bear to think about it, but now I would say to any woman in that situation, "Ask yourself whether you are going to accept that you've been abused for x number of years, and you can't do anything about it except go. Or whether you are going to ignore it and live the rest of your life caught in this pattern. *The rest of your life.*"'

The first step for an abused woman is to recognise what is happening to her, that she has the right to be happy and live in safety, and that her partner's controlling behaviour is unacceptable. Remember that domestic abuse and coercive control are crimes. And it is particularly important that women who are being psychologically, socially, financially and verbally ill-treated by their partners should understand that they are just as abused as women who are attacked with hammers and knives – and, furthermore, they do not have to put up with it.

Five out of the six women who have told of their experiences in this book have left their husbands and boyfriends and, to varying degrees, have begun to rebuild their self-esteem and their lives – often slowly, painfully and with very mixed emotions. But they have all – with help from friends, relations and counsellors – found a way forward.

## 'Are you abused and controlled by your partner?'

To all women who feel unhappy, trapped, isolated and controlled in their relationships, ask yourself some searching questions.

- Are you afraid of your partner? Do you feel you have to change your behaviour to please him – for example, do you avoid challenging him, or doing and saying things which might make him angry? Perhaps you tell white lies to avoid his temper, so that little things such as lying about whom you are talking to on the phone become instinctive.
- Do you appear confident and self-assured at work and with your friends but nervous and afraid to express an opinion when he is around?
- Has your partner ever threatened you, or intimidated you by using violent language or smashing up the furniture?
- Do you feel you have no hobbies or friends of your own? Does your partner make it difficult for you to see family and friends? Does he expect you to be with *him* all the time? Is he jealous or possessive?
- Do you find yourself agreeing with his criticisms of your friends and others? Do you adopt his values and attitudes simply to preserve the peace?
- Does he exclude you from his life? Does he seem secretive? Does he find excuses not to take you places such as office parties or to meet his friends and colleagues?
- Is he chauvinistic? Does he work all hours, yet insist that no wife of his is going to work? Or if you do work, is he jealous of what you do (irrespective of the fact that the family may rely on the money you earn)? Is he suspicious of your colleagues – does he think they are coming between you and him, or unjustly accuse you of having an affair with someone at work?
- Does he insist that the home and the children are your responsibility, and refuse to help out, even if you both have full-time jobs?

- Does he get over-involved in your life, solving all your problems in a seemingly caring way, such as getting your car repaired, filling in your tax forms, sorting out your car insurance, making all your decisions for you – until he has undermined your independence?

- Does he frequently humiliate and embarrass you, show you up or put you in the wrong – often in front of family and friends – so that you feel that *he* gets all the sympathy, and *you* are seen in a bad light?

- Do you feel that whatever you do you cannot seem to please him – that you cannot seem to win?

- Does he constantly bring up past 'misdemeanours' as if he is keeping a mental diary of everything you have done 'wrong' to use against you later? Do you feel as though he is always trying to catch you out?

- Does he lie, even about small things? Is he demanding, childish? Is he a perfectionist to the point of being petty about small things?

- Does he operate on double standards? Does he, for example, demand that you do everything according to his idea of an orderly, regimented timetable, while he does things when he feels like it?

- Do you always find you *have to* put him first and yourself last? Do you juggle a job with a family, exhausting yourself in the process, while he pursues outside interests? It may be that this pattern is so ingrained that you put yourself last in the subtlest, most unconscious ways. For example, do you say things like 'He's very good, he lets me go out with my friends once a week.' Think about it – what you are really saying is: he *allows* me to do these things. What he is doing, in fact, is *controlling* you.

- Does he expect you to be his emotional prop, yet fail to give you the same kind of attention, accusing you of being oversensitive or self-centred – when in fact he is being the self-centred one? Have there been times when you have needed understanding and affection – perhaps when a close relative or friend is ill or has died – only to be asked, 'But what about me – I was close to them too' or 'I wish you'd spend as much time worrying about *me*'?

- Does he always turn conversations around to centre on himself? Is it always *me, me, me*?
- Is he narcissistic? Does he always have to win? To be perfect? Always right? Does he constantly criticise and blame you or others for everything that is wrong in his life, rather than accept that he might have made a mistake?
- Is making love a shared, intimate experience, or do you feel that he is simply using your body without any consideration for your feelings?
- Do you sometimes doubt your judgement – or even your sanity? Do you feel guilty that you are unhappy? Do you feel that you must be to blame if things are going wrong – and does your partner imply that this is the case?
- If you leave, or threaten to leave, does he become all charming again and rush back into your life? Does he start telling *you* how special you are and then when you are attached to him again does he resort to his abusive behaviour?

If a woman recognises her relationship in this checklist, she is being controlled and abused – she may not necessarily have bruises to show for it, but emotional abuse can be just as debilitating.

### *How to recognise emotional abuse*
The following examples will also help you to recognise emotional abuse. Does your partner say:

- You're crazy. I'll have you sectioned.
- You're hysterical. No one will believe you.
- You couldn't possibly manage without me. You'd never cope on your own.
- Nobody else would have you. You can't cope with a real relationship.

- You're a slag/whore/bitch/tart/slut.
- You look awful. You've got a terrible body.
- You're mad/you're loony.
- Leave if you want to, but how do you think you will live?
- I'm telling you – you and the kids will be on the street.
- You won't get any benefits.
- If you divorce me, you won't get custody of the children.
- I'll tell social services you are a drug addict/alcoholic/liar/ unfit mother.
- If you leave me, my career will be ruined and it'll be all your fault.
- If you divorce me, I will make sure you don't get a penny.
- If you leave me, I'll kill myself.
- If you try to escape, I'll kill you and the children.
- If you try anything, I'll have you deported.
- You leave, and I'll come after you and beat your brains out.
- I'll tell your friends/family/boss what a bad wife you are.
- If you leave, I'll kidnap the children and take them abroad.

If your partner says any of these things to you, then you are being emotionally abused.

Facing up to the fact that you are abused can be bewildering, confusing and frightening, as Melinda found out. 'When I actually said those words, "I am abused", I felt stupid, as if I had been made a fool of,' she says. 'I was an independent, intelligent person – how could this have happened to me? And why didn't I see it earlier? But one of the best things that counselling did for me was to show me that I wasn't stupid and that Trevor's behaviour was actually nothing to do with me. It was his problem.' It is hard to recognise abuse because Charm Syndrome Man's behaviour changes insidiously. The abuse creeps so gradually into the relationship that often a woman cannot see what is happening.

Women in Melinda's situation have enough to cope with without making things harder by blaming themselves and feeling silly or guilty for having lived with an abusive man. It is just like finding themselves the victims of a hijack – it could happen to anyone. But, unlike hijackings, abusive relationships are both prevalent and kept secret. Their existence, and their extent, need to be exposed.

When I am counselling women I often use another analogy. I tell them: imagine you are riding a tiger in the jungle. It's dangerous to stay put but if you get off, the tiger may eat you. So what do you do? It feels as though you are in a no-win situation. But there is an alternative. You could try grabbing the branches which are all around you, and pull yourself off, out of his reach. Eventually – and sadly – he will pursue someone else, and you will feel safe and confident enough to plant your feet back on the ground.

It is time to be positive and grab some of those branches: reach out to other people, build your self-esteem, find new interests. Give yourself credit for recognising the situation *now*, and for wanting to do something about it. Rather than waste your strength on negative feelings, you need to congratulate yourself on having coped for so long. It takes tremendous strength to live with manipulation, control and abuse every day, while maintaining any semblance of ordinary life.

Often it helps to talk to someone who will listen, understand and help.

### 'Tell someone...'

The first thing to do is talk to somebody you can trust,' says Rebecca. 'I know it's an old cliché, but a problem shared is a problem halved. Coming to Refuge and speaking to someone was the turning point for me. So I think it's so important to talk to someone who understands and maybe also has a professional understanding. Having said that,' she admits, 'the hardest thing was telling somebody first of all. When I first rang Refuge I felt that you would say, "You can't come here, you're not a battered wife. You're supposed to have broken bones and things." I really thought that.'

When Rebecca first came to see me, like many women she did not really think of herself as abused. She only knew that she was unhappy. Often I ask such women to imagine what they would say if their best friend came to them and told them the same story. How would they react if they discovered that their best friend's partner was abusing her in all sorts of ways? Wouldn't they tell her that it was not her fault, that he had no right to behave in that way, that she is a worthwhile person and does not deserve such treatment? Often it helps women to distance themselves in this way. They are able to see things much more clearly if they imagine their problems as belonging to someone else.

A woman should not feel that if she asks for help she has failed in her relationship, or that she is betraying her partner because she cannot take the abuse anymore. Keeping her problems to herself will only help to perpetuate the abuse – both on an individual level and for women throughout society.

Talking to the *right* person is important. Though it may be that a woman will benefit from talking to someone with the professional skills to show her a way forward, just talking to a friend can be the first step for many women. Often the first reaction is going to be disbelief. Be prepared for reactions like 'I can't believe it – he's so brilliant, so charming' or 'We all thought you were quite happy.' But if such friends are really going to be supportive, once they have got over the shock they will listen, believe what a woman says and not judge or blame her.

However, if they refuse to accept that the man could behave in this way, if they say things like 'Why don't you go out and buy a sexy nightie?' or 'Go away for a weekend' or 'Cook him a candle-lit dinner' (the sort of crass options suggested in women's magazines in articles with headlines like 'How To Win Your Man Back'), then a woman needs to turn to someone else who can be more constructive – someone who will listen and not blame her, who will encourage and help her to see that she has options; someone who will understand that she is swimming in a sea of despair, guilt, shame, fear. She herself needs to accept that she has already expended prodigious efforts to make the relationship work – it is not she who needs to change, but her partner.

Opening up about her fears to the right person makes them more manageable, so it becomes easier for her to cope with her anxieties. Just talking about her experiences can make her feel much stronger, less guilty. Once things are out in the open she may be able to see her situation more clearly, to see that her husband or boyfriend has no justification for treating her in this way, and that there are alternatives – and people who will help her to achieve them.

A good first step to accessing support is visiting Refuge's website (**www.refuge.org.uk**). However, if a woman is concerned her abuser is monitoring her internet usage, her safest option would be to access the internet from somewhere like a trusted friend's house, an internet café or local library. There is also the National Domestic Violence Helpline, run by Refuge and Women's Aid, which is open 24 hours a day, seven days a week. Specialist advisers are there to give women support and information about what their options are in the short and long term.

It is important for a woman to build up her own supporting network: sympathetic friends, support groups, therapists – whoever she can trust and call upon when she has doubts and fears and her resolve is weakening and she feels tempted to make excuses for her partner. Hazel says, 'I'd advise women in my situation to confide in somebody and go for help. I know it's hard, but they mustn't think they're the only ones it's happened to, they shouldn't feel dirty or unclean. Go for help, because if you don't it doesn't get better. It gets worse. I believe that once somebody has abused you that way for a long time, it won't change. If you want any kind of life, I think you've got to realise that you have to be away from your abuser. Life is too short to live like that. Just talk about it. Tell people.'

Laura was put in a position where she had to tell complete strangers about her situation, but she found that opening up about it in this way can be a good form of therapy. She explains, 'Because James had gone to the children's headmaster and headmistress and said things like "My wife's crazy, my wife's drunk, and my wife's a drug addict, she's irresponsible and she's thrown me out of the house and is living in an immoral way taking drugs with somebody else", I had to do things like go to them and say, "Look, I'm not an alcoholic."

'I had to put my case to these people I'd never met before, and I had to learn to go there, be calm, be me, and say what the facts were, when I was actually trembling and shaking and feeling far less like me than I'd ever felt in my life. And it was very difficult indeed at first. But, gradually, people have got to know me, and they are very supportive to me. But at first I could tell that they were just sort of testing, and that's very tough when you're going through all of that.

'I must say that both the headmaster and the headmistress were wonderful. The minute I said, "Well, actually the problem was that he used to hit me", they were both fantastic. They said, "Well done, you've obviously done the right thing", which was amazing. Had they said, "I don't believe you", it would have been devastating – because there had been a lot of that, mostly from people connected with him and his family, who believed his side of the story and nothing else. And because I had to face that with so many different people in entirely different situations, including courts and solicitors and everything else, it became therapeutic in itself.

'It was like that with friends too. Because they didn't really know the situation – because I had never told them – they would ring up and say, "Look, why have you left him? He's desperate and he's going to commit suicide", and so I'd have to go through the whole story again, and each time a bit more would come out. And it was good to talk about it. It's just the fact of saying, "Look, I've done it. I've walked away. I don't have to put up with it, and I won't." By doing that, you can fight your way through.'

### 'Take your time'

'After I had talked to people and finally admitted what was happening, I had an overwhelming feeling of panic,' says Melinda. 'Okay, I had said those words, "I am abused", but now what? I felt that I couldn't stay in the relationship, now that I could see what was going on. But the idea of leaving, of finding somewhere to go, of making all those decisions terrified me. I think that, despite everything, I wasn't ready to leave. The emotional bond with Trevor was still very strong.'

'You have to make your own decision. If somebody tells you you've got to leave, it doesn't help you,' agrees Hazel, who also found the idea of simply packing her bags and walking out on Jimmy forever too much to face in one fell swoop.

It is very, very important for a woman to make her own decisions in her own time. She should try not to feel overwhelmed by the need to answer the question, 'Should I stay or should I leave?' And well-meaning friends and advisers should never try to force her into leaving. The last thing she wants to do is swap one person who is controlling her life for another friend or relative who appears to be doing the same thing, however well-intentioned. It is time for the woman to take her own decisions, to begin to regain control over her *own* life, however slow that process may be.

Many women, who tell me they would like to leave their partner, obviously half hope that there is some pithy formula with almost magical powers which will enable them to walk painlessly away from the relationship. They feel paralysed. But leaving a partner is more of a process than a single decisive act. I always suggest to women trapped in this way that they try asking themselves what is the worst thing that could happen if they leave. Many women say they are afraid of being lonely, or they worry about taking the children away from their father, or they feel that they will not find another man. Sometimes they worry about managing financially. Then I suggest they ask themselves if these fears outweigh the misery of staying. Perhaps there are other alternatives they haven't considered.

Look at your life as impersonally as you can, and be honest with yourself. It is probable that you already feel lonely and isolated. And will your children really be better off staying in an unhappy home?

You worry about not finding another man, but right now you are feeling worthless and unloved. Your self-esteem is low – it is only natural to think that no one else will want you. But as you begin to see that you are not alone, that you are not to blame and that you are an important, worthwhile person, all that will change. Once you have regained your independence, you may even decide that you do not want another relationship for a while.

Leaving may be taking a step into the unknown, but that unknown may be far more fulfilling than your life as it is. Ask yourself what you really want from life and how you think you can best achieve it: by going or by staying? Melinda could not forget the good side of her relationship with Trevor, but I asked her to weigh up the good times and the bad times and see where the balance lay. I wanted her to try to work out in percentage terms how much of her life was happy and how much was unhappy. Exploring all these questions put her on the road to change. But it took time – three years, in fact – before she made the break for good.

'Once a fortnight I'd say, "This relationship has got to finish. I don't want it anymore,"' she says. 'Then we'd get into this cycle where I would leave – or he would leave – and then we'd try again. He'd be very, very apologetic, incredibly comforting. And I'd go along with that. I wanted to be comforted. And I missed him. Still do – the charming, nice side, that is.'

Most women I talk to try to leave many times. They often say to me, 'I knew I should leave – but there were just too many obstacles in my way.' As we have seen, women are often terribly trapped and frightened, so it is little wonder that it takes a great deal of time and courage for them to summon the strength to go. And, as Melinda points out, they have no reason to feel guilty about that: 'I think that, when you are so confused, the leaving process is not something that happens quickly. Neither is it something that I think you should feel bad about when it doesn't happen, when you do cope.

'I think that, for me, going back all those times was part of the leaving process,' she says now. 'I had to keep doing it, because eventually, when I left for the last time, I knew that I had done everything I could. I knew I really wanted to leave and I knew why I was leaving. There was a stronger bond between us than I was aware of, and it was very hard. But I began to see that there was a definite pattern to his behaviour.

'He would flare up, get angry, hit or punch me – for no apparent reason. Then he would walk out, or I'd leave. I'd be very upset, but I would be quite firm. I would say to myself, "I've got to finish it. It's got to stop. I won't cope with it anymore." Just when I'd start to feel a bit stronger he'd come around and be very, very nice. It was quite insidious the way he would creep back into my life. He'd be very charming. We'd chat. Things would be very calm, and I'd start forgetting the bad times. That funny thing about memory would start happening – when that whole sweet, loving side of him came through I just got sucked in again.

'I'd go through a period of feeling pretty bad because in a way I had failed, but also I felt relieved as well, and I enjoyed the good parts, because there were a lot of good parts. But what happened in the end was I started to feel unsafe when he was being nice. A voice inside me started to say, "This isn't real. Okay, it's nice, but the niceness is a forerunner to abuse. And I know that's coming next." And that was horrible. That was when I started to face up to the abuse. The objective part of me that said "I'm not going to accept this" came through more and more.

'Gradually, each time I left, I found I went back with less of me. There was a bigger part each time which remained separate – rational, I suppose. I became more skilful about speaking my mind. My objective self came through, the side that kept saying "I'm not going to accept this relationship". But it was still hard. Each time I left I tried to be strong, and say, "This is it." But one part of me would say, "Come on. You tried to leave before and you failed."

'The last time I went back to him I'd been away for six months and hadn't even looked at him – but I still went back. I shocked myself. But when I went back that last time, it was virtually a formal relationship. We had nothing in common. I was so cautious. I remember he shouted at me, "You won't even let me get angry with you anymore." That last attempt was so unsuccessful that I had no doubts at all about leaving for good, and I think perhaps I went back just to convince myself of that.'

For most women who leave, there is a turning point, and for every woman it is different. Laura endured everything, from bruises to sexual abuse – including James's infidelity – but what finally made her snap was when he hit her in front of the children. 'I finally said, "Right, that's it,"' she recalls. 'I'd got to the point where I didn't care how I was going to do it, but I was going to leave. I'd just had it. All I figured was: "This is terrifying, this is frightening, this is bad, and this is killing me, and I can't do it anymore."

'What really gave me the strength to stick to it was that just before it happened he had gone away with this woman he was seeing, and he had actually left me on my own for a couple of weeks and I had time to think, "Well, this isn't so bad – this is actually a better alternative than being frightened all the time. I would rather have some peace and be on my own." And so when he came round to sort of try and persuade me that it would all be all right again, I was tearful, but I never once wavered and thought, "Let's try it again." I just knew I couldn't put up with it not working again. I just didn't have the strength to try again – that was the difference. And I also realised that I *could* be without him.'

### 'I can't leave'

When Rebecca weighed up her situation, she felt that she simply could not walk out on Ralph, at least until the children were old enough to leave home. 'After talking to counsellors and friends,' she says, 'I woke up to what Ralph was doing. I could see that all the things he did that drove me mad fitted into his need to control. But I still loved him. And he had never been violent. I wasn't scared of him, just worn down by it all.

'Once I accepted that I was abused, I knew that I *could* leave, and in a way that made me feel less trapped. I knew I had the strength to do it, but I felt that if I could make small changes, bit by bit, make him see that he couldn't grind me down with his moods and his insistence on making all the decisions, then I might be able to make it work. The important thing was that by *deciding* to stay, rather than feeling I had no option, I felt as if I had got some control back into my life.'

Many women, like Rebecca, are unable to leave their partners – because of the children, because they have nowhere to go and no money, because they are too scared, or because they simply cannot give up on the relationship. Other women leave briefly, but return after a period of separation.

Abused women find it hard to leave their partners because, understandably, they have become emotionally dependent on them. They become extensions of their abusers. For an abused woman to lose her partner raises the frightening prospect of losing herself. So unless she can do something which will sever the emotional dependency between herself and her partner, it is unlikely that she will leave him.

It is important not to feel guilty for needing Charm Syndrome Man so much. It can be all too easy to fall for someone as energetic and exciting as Charm Syndrome Man. To free yourself from him, you have to develop new interests, participate in new activities and find new friends. Inch your way along slowly. You do not need him to be fulfilled. As one abused woman has put it: 'Don't worry, don't panic. You won't die. You won't be alone forever. Leaving may be the hardest thing to do, but don't feel tempted to call him and start things all over again. He may be charming and wonderful at first, but then he will go back to his old behaviour. Call a friend, do some spring cleaning, go to the theatre, get drunk, but do not call him. The feelings of panic will pass. The pain gets less and less over time. Embarking on a new life is difficult, but you can do it.'

When abused women ask me for advice on how to cope, I tell them to remember that they will not change their partners (only their partners can do that). But they can alter their own responses to the abuse. The most important thing – as Rebecca realised – is to regain some kind of *control* over their lives.

I told Rebecca, 'Hard as it may be, try not to take his insults and abuse personally. Try to be objective. You know by now that his behaviour has nothing to do with you. It is his problem. Remind yourself you are not a slag and a whore, a lousy cook, a bad mother, a selfish self-centred hussy. Remember that when you first met him he told you that you were loving, clever, caring, fun to be with. You haven't changed – after all he still says such things during the phases when he isn't being abusive.'

I continued to see Rebecca regularly and she told me: 'I don't let Ralph's moods get to me anymore. When he is insulting I try to pretend that what he is saying has nothing to do with me. He called me a stupid fool the other night because I'd ruined the dinner, but I just reminded myself that he was doing it to make me feel small and to make himself seem better.

'Previously I would have been feeling guilty for being stupid and inadequate, but now I tell myself that that is *his* view of things, not mine. The more I can reject his opinions of me, the less he is able to hurt me. I feel much stronger, much more confident because of it. I feel active rather than passive. I tell myself that it isn't okay for anybody to treat me the way Ralph does at times. No one has the right to dictate to you, to undermine you in front of other people.'

Though Rebecca was now able to challenge Ralph mentally, it was important for her – and for other women in her situation – to realise that physically challenging her abuser, or even trying to argue with him, will not help. It can be dangerous if he is a violent man. Every woman has to judge for herself just how far she can show her independence before her life becomes more miserable or more unsafe than before. It is important to remember that even if Charm Syndrome Man loses one round, he will win the next –

because he makes the rules. He will simply start a new row or find another excuse to be abusive. He will argue until the small hours of the morning if necessary. He will not listen to his partner's point of view, or accept it.

It is far more constructive for a woman in Rebecca's situation to use her energy to build up her sense of self-worth than to waste it trying to change her partner. 'Remind yourself,' I told her, 'that Ralph is irrational in his criticism. He will do anything to prove he is in control.'

Charm Syndrome Man is what he is, but his partner can try to undo some of his messages, and in doing so feel better about herself. If he criticises her, instead of apologising she could say, 'You may be right' or 'I can see why you might be angry.' This tactic does not let him win (her first response implies, 'But you could be wrong!'); it is a way of possibly defusing the situation by denying him the chance to have an argument. It is a way of doing something positive, of taking control over the situation – whereas if she apologises and tries to justify herself, *he* remains in control.

It may seem such a small shift of emphasis, but it is quite a triumph for an abused woman to be able to say to herself, 'I am calling the shots here – he may not know it, but the fact is I am *choosing* to let him have his own way, rather than being bullied into it.'

I suggested to Rebecca that she could widen her interests and make new friends. Ralph might have a grumble and then forget about it – he might not even notice, some of the time. However, he might feel threatened by what he sees as her striking a blow for independence. What Rebecca had to decide for herself was just how far she could go before his negative reaction outweighed the advantages for her.

I also wanted Rebecca to know that she could always leave at some future point. And she did not have to wait for some incident which would make her feel justified in doing so. It would be enough to say, 'I've had enough' or 'I am unhappy.' No woman should ever feel she needs an excuse to leave.

A woman can plan for that day – if and when it happens – by doing little things, such as arranging for a friend to look after the children if she has to leave suddenly, keeping the number of the National Domestic Violence Helpline (run in partnership between Refuge and Women's Aid) handy, saving some money, even keeping a suitcase packed. She could improve her skills so that if she needs to get a job she is better equipped, or she could see a solicitor to find out what her rights would be if she decides to leave her partner. Then, if she does leave, she can do so from a position of strength.

### 'It's knowing you're not alone'

When women come to Refuge they are amazed to discover that they are not alone: that the confusing emotions they experience are shared by many, many women, who have similar stories to tell and can offer them a sense of comradeship – whether they remain with their partners or leave them.

'If you knew you had somebody to support you, you might come to the decision to leave a lot earlier,' says Beverley. 'Because that's all you want, somebody who you can rely on who will support you, and help you through it. Not necessarily financial support, but emotional support. Because it's very frightening going to court, and the police coming and people talking about you – that's one of the hardest things to deal with. I mean we're all social creatures, and nobody likes being talked about badly.'

Hazel says, 'When you get to the stage where you know you *can* leave, you need support. For a long time I was in a terrible state. I was so frightened. I phoned the Samaritans one night because I was going to kill myself. Everything seemed to get on top of me. I felt so lonely – even now I feel lonely sometimes. But I can cope with it, because the support is there.

'The hardest thing was that always, in the back of my mind, I was thinking, "What is he going to do? Is he ever going to let me go? Would he suddenly come back? Would he spring up in the middle of the night, and do something awful? Would he kidnap the kids?"

And then things started changing. I don't know exactly when they changed, but the support was always there when I needed it.'

As Rebecca says, 'It doesn't matter whether you leave your partner or you stay, you still need to know that there is a lifeline out there, that there are people who can put you on the right track again, if you start to get despondent.'

### 'You have to get in touch with your feelings'

When a woman has lived with an abusive man, she will usually have been so caught up in a web of guilt and insecurity that she suppresses her real feelings. Now it is time to begin to acknowledge them, however painful. A woman fleeing violence has lost her lover, her hopes and dreams, her home, belongings, familiar surroundings and people and financial security. She has suffered the loss of her bodily integrity and other less visible griefs, such as the beliefs she once had about herself and relationships. Until she is able to get in touch with those feelings and work through the pain and grief, she will not be able to act. If a woman is unsure of her feelings, how can she decide what she wants to do?

Sally says, 'When I was with Guy it seemed safer and easier to deny my feelings, but when we finally split up I faced up to how confused and angry and sad I was, instead of hiding all that. Once you admit to those feelings at least you can try to do something about them.'

Unsettling as it may seem, to be able to say things like 'I am frightened of the future,' rather than pretending that everything is okay, is the first step towards the new options open to a woman.

Rebecca found that getting in touch with her feelings was the first step towards distancing herself from Ralph's abuse. 'When he had said something particularly wounding, I made myself think, "How do I feel? Am I sad, angry, hurt, despairing?" Doing that made me less anxious, because I could see the effect his behaviour had on me, and I could take steps to alter my reactions.'

### 'You can't change him'

Melinda explains, 'The man will say, "If only you don't do this or that, our relationship will be better." But it *won't* be. No matter what you do, it will be wrong. You can go over hurdles trying to change things. But unless *he* is prepared to change, nothing will change.'

Laura says, 'I knew what was happening was wrong, always. But I wanted him without the violence. I wanted someone he wasn't. I thought I could love him out of it, make him happy, or whatever. And I couldn't. It just got worse and worse and worse. The more I put up with it, the worse it got. I put up with so much, making excuses, hoping it was going to work out.

'When I finally left, I'd tried and tried and *tried* to make it work – I felt as if I'd been doing all the trying and nobody else had, and it was just too late for him to turn round and say, "Let's do it again." And, in fact, looking back, I know bloody well that it would have just gone wrong again.'

In order to move forward, what an abused woman must ultimately accept is that nothing she does can alter the situation as it is – only he can change it, by facing up to his problem and genuinely wanting to change. And the hard fact is Charm Syndrome Man rarely wants to change. He will do everything he can to remain in charge, whether that means attacking his partner physically, emotionally, verbally, socially or psychologically. Just as she is the way she is, he is what he is. It is no use hoping that his charming loving side will one day reappear and stay. His behaviour will always be unpredictable. A woman cannot mould a man into something that he is not.

If she asks herself, 'Does altering my behaviour stop the abuse? If I am sure to cook his dinner on time, if I dress the way he likes, if I avoid inviting family around when he is there, does it have any effect on his behaviour?' the answer is almost certainly no.

Instead of using her emotional reserves to change and appease him, an abused woman can use her energy in a much more positive way: by focusing on her own needs and interests, and building her own identity. She has the right to be upset by her partner's behaviour, however much she may still care for him. It may not be advisable to object to his face, but she can assert herself in small ways which boost her self-esteem and help her regain confidence. Changing the woman's behaviour cannot change *his* behaviour, but what she can do is begin to take control of her own life.

### 'It's not your fault'

'All the time, when I was living with Dave,' says Beverley, 'some instinct was telling me, "You don't deserve this. This isn't right, it isn't your fault", but every other part of me was saying the opposite.'

'It is so important to remember that the things that are being done to you are not your fault. They are not of your making,' says Melinda. 'I had no reason to feel guilty. It was Trevor – and my family, who wouldn't believe what I was going through – who made me feel that way.'

Accepting that it is not her fault is a vital step for any woman. As long as she blames herself, her abuser has no need to own up to his behaviour, and she will never be able to stop trying to make things better within the relationship.

A woman has to learn to forgive herself for her shortcomings. Everyone has them. Her faults have nothing whatsoever to do with his abuse. She does not cause it. He chooses to behave in that way. Even if he has affairs, she needs to tell herself that Charm Syndrome Man will frequently stray no matter how 'perfect' she is, because he must always boost his macho image. It is natural to feel that in some way she must have driven him to it – because she was not attentive enough, she was not good enough in bed or she had 'let herself go' – but as long as she crucifies herself with these self-accusations she will never be able to find a way forward.

It is important for an abused woman to free herself from the kind of downward spiral of guilt in which Melinda found herself. Every little blow to her self-esteem made her feel more and more guilty, sapping her energy as she tried to make things work. Then when they didn't she felt guiltier than ever.

As she puts it, 'I used to feel guilty when Trevor criticised me. He made me feel guilty because the marriage wasn't working. So I spent all that time putting him first and myself last, and letting my friends go – and then all he did was lose interest in me, because he said I didn't make myself attractive enough for him, and I was boring because I never did anything. The result was that I felt even more guilty.'

Many women are confused because, whatever they do, their partners make them feel that they have failed. They believe that their failure to reach 'happy ever after' is due to some defect in themselves. As one woman said, 'I have always been outspoken and independent. I know I can be strong-willed, but I was like that when we met. And he used to say that was what he liked about me: that I had a mind of my own. So why does he put me down every time I say what I think? How come he wants me to be a different person now? Why does he make me feel guilty all the time?'

The irony is that Charm Syndrome Man *is* attracted to women who have such qualities. But once he is in a relationship he feels threatened by the very attributes he fell for in the first place. Now, if she behaves in a strong, independent way, he feels threatened, and scared that she might leave him. So he undermines her personality. He makes her feel unattractive, worthless – and guilty, because she thinks she has failed him. She feels she has lost her identity – and her marriage. Other people, outside the relationship, give her similar messages, and the spiral of guilt continues.

A woman needs to recognise that her partner is controlling her in this way because (however unconsciously) he wants to feel bigger and better than her. He may say that everything which goes wrong is her fault, he may say that she has personality problems, that if she changed her attitude everything would be okay – but what he is doing is manipulating and controlling her through guilt. And while he is able to do so, she will be unable to act for herself.

The way out of this cycle of guilt is to start devoting time to herself, putting her own needs and desires to the top of the list, for a change.

### 'You have to think of yourself as a real and worthwhile person again'

'I think women definitely need therapy and counselling afterwards, because for so long you've been told that you are dirt. You can't just wave a wand and become a real person again,' said Hazel.

It is important for a woman to take one day at a time, to try to make decisions at her own speed. She could congratulate herself on each small success. For so long she has been denied the right to think of herself as a worthwhile person. Now it is time to try to look at things through new eyes, to be positive about herself, to say, 'I am important. It's time to pay attention to *me*. The very fact that I have coped for so long means that I am a strong person.'

She could tell herself, 'I am only human, it is normal to "make mistakes".' Or 'From now on I make my own decisions and, whether they are right or wrong, I'm not going to feel guilty about them. It is *my* life, and I don't have to live up to anyone else's expectations.'

Instead of looking back and saying, 'If only I had done such and such', she could try to make a list of the ways in which her partner tries to control her. Once they are written down in black and white they may help her to see the situation more clearly and understand what he has been trying to do.

She could make another list of all the things she would like to achieve in the next three years, as a way of focusing on herself rather than her partner.

In a third list she could try to note all her positive qualities – however silly they may sound, they may make her feel better about herself. If she has all these good things going for her, she does not deserve to be so unhappy.

Making such lists is not trivial: the idea is to enable the woman to distance herself from her situation and see it clearly and objectively.

Re-establishing contact with people outside the relationship and breaking the isolation so many women feel is another important step in building self-esteem, because it will help an abused woman to realise that she is not as dependent on her partner as she may think. Women grow up believing that they need a man to look after them. So it is often hard to say, 'I can be myself. I can be independent.' But developing her own identity and assuming control over her own life is vital for a woman if she is going to free herself from the influence of her abusive partner.

Sally says, 'All the time I was with Guy I felt that my happiness depended on him. When we split up I felt lost at first, but now the wonderful thing is that I don't have to depend on any man to make me feel good about myself. No man can actually do that for you, you have to really like yourself first. Yes, it would be nice to meet someone else – as long as he didn't behave like Guy! – but I don't feel any pressure on me to have another relationship. I have other friendships, I go to the theatre, I read. I do all the things I couldn't do because he always wanted me to do something else. No way am I sitting around waiting for Mr Right to come along.'

That is not to suggest that the answer to everything is to substitute an abusive partner with a flurry of work and partying. That does not build self-esteem either. People often bury themselves in their work to cover up pain, loneliness, inadequacy and a host of other problems, but work only acts like sticking plaster: it covers up the wounds, it does not heal them.

## *How do you recognise low self-esteem?*

- Do you hear yourself saying:
  - 'I should have done...'
  - 'I ought to have said...'
  - 'If only I had...'
- Do you constantly apologise?
- Are you indecisive?

- Do you doubt your own judgement?
- Do you worry about what others will think of you?
- Are you confident when you are at work or with friends but at home you find that events and feelings are out of your control?
- Do you say 'yes' when you would really rather say 'no'?
- Do you feel that nobody could like you?
- Do you wish you were someone else?

If you answered 'yes' to any of these questions, you are undervaluing yourself. Living with abuse can erode a woman's self-esteem and leave her feeling very vulnerable.

Real self-esteem is about accepting yourself – warts and all – and being your own best friend. You do not have to become the head of a company, climb Everest or be seen in the hottest nightclubs to be important and worthwhile. Just 'being' is enough. Go your own way, find your own style. Just because the world seems to be saying, 'Be sexy' or 'Be a power dresser' or whatever is fashionable at the moment, does not mean you have to follow suit. If you do, you are acting, you are not being true to yourself. It might be fun to be sexy or powerful, but if it is not *you* then it will not give you any real sense of self-worth. A person with real self-esteem would say: 'It may be fun to be sexy' or 'How fascinating to have all that power' or 'Isn't it interesting that people are all so different?' or 'But I am what I am' or 'I'll go my own way.'

It is not easy building self-esteem when you live with a man who abuses you day in day out. Over time a woman begins to believe the negative things her partner says about her, and very often he is so controlling that she finds it impossible to focus on her own needs. However, as Rebecca found, doing small things which made her feel good about herself helped enormously, even if it was only taking a swim, having a manicure or listening to music. It is important for a woman to inch herself along slowly. She can try telling herself that she is not stupid or lazy and so on. Whether she stays with the relationship or leaves, she can build her self-esteem by doing things like cooking a nice meal, for *herself*, fantasising about a future in which she is happy, visiting a friend, having her hair done, remembering times when she felt loved and fulfilled, taking some form of exercise, meditating or contacting friends with whom she has lost touch.

As Laura says, 'It is so important to get completely away from the idea of the abuse, and do things for yourself, strengthen your contacts with other people and do things that you enjoy doing, that make you feel good and give you security – become involved in the outside world again.'

## 'You have to let out all the anger'

'For about two weeks after I left Trevor for the last time,' says Melinda, 'I felt the most intense anger towards him. I was consumed with anger. I started thinking about all the things that had happened and I felt very, very indignant. I relived it all and I felt I had been absolutely powerless. I thought, "How dare he do all those things?" I wanted to punish him. I wanted revenge. It was awful. I was obsessed and I didn't like those feelings. But after two weeks the feelings suddenly diminished, and I began to feel more separate from him. Once the anger had gone, I felt as if something had broken between us. I felt able to look towards the future without being so tied up with this man.'

Using anger constructively can play a vital part in strengthening a woman's resolve to free herself from her abusive partner. For so long she will have internalised her anger and her pain, unable to express her frustrations for fear of sparking off more abuse. Bottling up anger in that way can lead to stress and depression. It can often result in a woman taking it out on her children, friends and colleagues.

Being angry is a good sign. It is another way of showing that she is getting in touch with her feelings again, after years of suppressing them. Just telling people, 'I am angry about what he has done,' or saying, 'I am important. He has no right to treat me like this' is a way forward.

A woman needs to know that she is not to blame for the abuse, that it is her partner's problem, not hers. Once she can accept that, she can see that she does not deserve her treatment and she can feel justified in being angry. And constructive anger plays an important part in rebuilding a woman's self-esteem.

Whether a woman leaves her partner or stays with him, breaking Charm Syndrome Man's control over her is hard. There will be times when she will falter – and, if she leaves, she may be tempted to go back to what is familiar, however unhappy that life may be.

However, if a woman can accept the reality of her situation and let go of the 'happy ever after' fantasy – the belief that she can somehow turn her partner permanently into the reliable, loving and tender man she thought she had found – then she can channel that energy into creating a new life for herself, one in which she can find true meaning and fulfilment.

A woman can change the way she feels and use her energy to make a positive change in her situation by remembering the following:

- Overcoming abuse is a gradual process and can be taken one step at a time – you do not have to take decisions until you are ready.
- Carefully considering each option in turn will give you the confidence to get a grip on the situation, whereas getting stuck on the whole question 'Should I stay or leave?' can be overwhelming.
- Even if you are not perfect, your partner is not entitled to abuse you.
- Finding a solution takes time, but it is possible.

An abused woman *can* do it. As five of our six women can testify, there is life after Charm Syndrome Man.

## For men

I would love to be able to tell you that Jimmy, Guy, Ralph and the other abusive men we have heard so much about throughout this book have admitted that their partners are not to blame, taken responsibility for their own behaviour and tried to change. But the truth is that, in terms of a way forward, abusive men have difficulty in facing reality. The very nature of Charm Syndrome Man prevents him from admitting that his behaviour is unacceptable. But unless all men – not just abusers – can wake up to the reality that controlling, dominating behaviour is abusive, that it cannot be justified as 'the way men are supposed to behave', then there will be no way forward.

Just as I asked women who are reading this book to look at their lives and their relationships and answer a few basic questions, I would like to appeal to their partners to do the same thing:

- Apart from physically hurting your wife or girlfriend, have you ever threatened to do it, or intimidated her by shouting, swearing, smashing up furniture or harming household pets, as if to imply, 'You could be next'?
- When you make love, are you still tender and loving, do you still want to make her feel special, or do you just satisfy yourself and forget about her?
- Have you ever made her have sex in a way that worried her? Or accused her of being frigid if she does not want to make love? Are there times when you have called her degrading names and abused her verbally, put her down or ignored her in front of other people, and ridiculed her?
- Do you forget that once you thought this woman was everything you ever wanted? That once you told her you loved her just the way she was? Now do you concentrate on her faults?
- If she challenges you on *anything*, do you accuse her of being a nag, always complaining, and ruining the relationship with her whinging?
- Have you ever come home from work to dinner and refused to eat it, telling her it is horrible – or even thrown it away?
- Once you have children, do you pretend they don't exist? Do you speak adoringly of them to others but at home fail to notice them or help to care for them?

- Do you use the idea that men and women have separate roles in order to avoid cooking, cleaning, washing up and looking after the children?
- Are you jealous and possessive? You may immediately answer no. But think about it. Do you try to change her life by preventing her from doing the things she wants to do, like going out with her girlfriends and seeing the people she wants to see? Do you open her mail?
- Do you make promises to your partner then let her down? Are you unpredictable? Do you refuse to go to social events at the last possible minute, leaving your partner to explain your absence to others?
- Do you accuse her of having affairs without any grounds? Or cover up for the fact that *you* are having an affair by saying that she must be paranoid?
- Have you ever tried to interfere with her relationship with the children – for example, sending them to bed on your return home, when you know she enjoys spending time with them, or tried to turn them against her by saying things like, 'Your mother is always spending too much' or 'Look what I have to put up with – she's always arguing with me'?
- Do you overrule her when it comes to making the decisions? Do you think that *you* know what makes her happy? How often does she have the say in what you do, where you go on holiday, what colour to paint the living room, when to switch off the TV?
- Do you decide how to spend the money – do you ration it out and expect your partner to account for every penny she has spent? Or do you feel entitled to spend *her* money?
- Do you confide in her, or do you exclude her from your feelings? Do you think that women should be intuitive and understanding, that therefore you have no need to talk to your partner? Have you become secretive, or do you actually lie to her?
- Do you expect her to understand, forgive, and look after all your emotional needs – without feeling that you have to reciprocate? Do you think that these are feminine, not masculine qualities?

- Have you ever decided to punish her for not behaving the way you think she should – for example, do you try to frighten her by showing your anger, or refuse to speak to her for days when you know she cannot stand your silence?
- If you are arguing with your wife or girlfriend, do you find it hard to concede that she might be right, or hard to accept criticism? Are you always on the defensive? Do you accuse *her* of changing – and tell her that is why you come home late from work so much, or go to the pub without her?
- Rather than accept that you might be in the wrong, do you try to shift the blame by saying things like 'You don't know what you're talking about – you've had too much to drink', when really you know she has only had one glass of wine?
- Do you constantly remind her of things she 'did wrong', and bring up old grievances whenever you get the opportunity?
- Take a look at other areas of your life too. Do you put other people down and criticise them, so that you appear in a better light? Do you blame other people for everything that goes wrong, such as colleagues at work, other drivers on the road?
- Do you have to win, to be the best: on the football pitch or the squash court? Do you want to be the centre of attention in the pub or at parties? Do you like to be seen as Mr Nice Guy – but forget to behave the same way with your partner?
- Do you have 'real' friends, to whom you can turn when you are in trouble, or have you cut yourself off from other people, expecting your partner to fulfil every emotional need?
- Have you ever threatened suicide, or vowed to hurt or kill her or the children if your partner says she is leaving you?
- Do you find it hard to express your fears, worries, sadness in any other way than anger or rage?
- Are you jealous about possessions, other than 'your woman': your car, stereo, etc?
- Do you make sexist jokes, and talk about women as 'bitches' or 'dumb blondes'?

Of course, no one has a perfect relationship. We all say things we do not mean, we wound the people we care about most, we make mistakes – but look at this list carefully. Do you see something more than a 'yes' to one or two questions? Do you recognise a pattern?

Does your partner complain about these things, has she left you for any of these reasons? Does she say she is frightened of you, or withdraw from you? Does your behaviour alienate her?

Have the children ever seemed wary, or asked, 'Why did you hurt Mummy?'

If the answer to any of these questions is 'yes', it means that you are involved in a pattern of controlling behaviour, which – whether you know it or not – you learned long before you ever set eyes on your partner. It is not something which just happened one day – this kind of behaviour is something which has been encouraged and nurtured throughout society for centuries, as I showed in Chapter 5. Abusive men have learned that it is their right to control and dominate women, if necessary through physical, emotional, financial or verbal abuse.

## 'Accept responsibility for what you are doing'

The first step for an abusive man – just as it is for an abused woman – is to face the truth. For the man, that means admitting that his behaviour is unacceptable and taking responsibility for his actions, rather than blaming his partner. Nothing that she does can cause him to behave the way that he does. It is no use hiding behind the explanatory myths, such as drink or drugs, stress or unemployment. These things may make him feel frustrated and angry, but they are only excuses – they do not cause the abuse. Many men have similar problems, but do not abuse their partners.

Abusive behaviour is not caused by your partner or problems in a relationship. Nor is it caused by drink, stress or mental illness. Abusive behaviour is about trying to maintain or gain power and control over your partner. As one man I appeared with on a television series on woman abuse admitted, 'You want control of your belongings. If you don't get what you want, you strike out. I have to have control around me totally so that I feel safe and adequate as a person...I never blamed myself. I might have been the assailant, but I never blamed myself. It was: "You made me hit you." It was never me.'

It is no use seeking any form of joint counselling, such as marital or couples' therapy, until a man can accept the basic fact that his behaviour is about control and he alone is responsible for it. It is not the relationship which must change, but *his* behaviour, and while he is still controlling and dominating his wife or girlfriend there is no chance of building trust or communicating properly.

Accepting responsibility is no guarantee that his abuse will stop, but understanding why a man behaves in the way he does is crucial. Stopping abuse is the goal – and that includes all forms of emotional abuse and controlling behaviour, as well as violence. And if the relationship ends, one way in which a man may accept his responsibility is to accept her decision to leave. He could respect restraining orders and pay maintenance without being grudging about it.

### 'You are not alone'

Abusive men are not alone; there are many men from all walks of life, social positions and income brackets who behave in a similar fashion. However, that is no excuse. The bottom line is: what they are doing is unacceptable.

It is against the law for a man to hit his partner, even if they are married and the assault takes place within the home. And it can lead to murder. Forty-four per cent of female homicide victims are killed by present or former male partners.[82] And while emotional and psychological abuse may not leave visible wounds it can drive a woman away, split the family and ruin everyone's lives just as surely as broken bones and bruises.

## 'You have a choice'

Violence is a learned behaviour. What is learned can be unlearned. Men always have a choice. Everywhere they look they may be bombarded with the idea that men are the leaders, the controllers, the breadwinners, and that women are less important. The history books set the precedent for men's power, and society promotes it in the home, in the workplace, in schools, in Parliament, in the media and in the way it denies resources to abused women. By facing up to his behaviour – and its causes – an abusive man may be going against everything he has been taught by society, his peers and even his family about masculinity and what it means to be a man.

An abusive man could explore *why* he has felt able to abuse his partner. Why doesn't she deserve the same respect he gives to male friends and colleagues? Not all men have to go along with these traditional views and attitudes (and many do not). They always have choices. They have the choice whether or not to accept those traditional attitudes towards men and women. And even if they accept them, they do not have to go so far as to abuse their partners to maintain their position. That is the second choice they make.

Their wives may be irritating, ignorant, unreasonable – no one is saying all women are angels. But a woman cannot *make* a man behave abusively. He always has an alternative. He can try to talk to her, see her point of view and not impose his views on her. As a last resort, he can walk away, go to the pub, call a friend. Or even get a divorce.

## 'Talk to people'

An abusive man who seriously wants to change can help himself by cultivating friends and contacts outside his relationship, rather than demanding that his partner meets every emotional need. Many men who feel depressed, worried and suicidal because of their behaviour find it difficult to talk to anyone close to them – they may feel ashamed, or unable to admit their abuse, even to themselves. But there are doctors, therapists or counsellors they could turn to, who will treat their cases in complete confidence.

An abusive man could start by talking to his GP, who can refer him for counselling, or contact a local men's group. Respect – the national association for domestic violence perpetrator programmes and associated support services – can help you find a programme.

If a man isolates himself from outsiders, he is more prone to possessiveness and jealousy, he will suffocate his partner with his dependency and his controlling behaviour, and become more and more abusive whenever he feels threatened by an act of independence.

A man could ask himself whether behaving jealously is going to achieve anything. Even if she *was* being unfaithful, would being jealous help anyone? It certainly doesn't entitle a man to use violence. Monitoring her life and interrogating her about her every movement will ultimately have the effect that he dreads most. It will drive her away.

### 'She has a right to her own life'

An abusive man must accept that his partner has a right to live her own life without being dominated and controlled. He has no right to 'keep her in line'. And living independent lives need not interfere with the intimacy of a relationship. Of course, people who live completely separate lives can drift apart, but the kind of dependency on which an abuser insists is just as destructive. There is a balance, in which both partners accept the right of the other to be their own people, have their own friends and activities, state their own opinions, yet are still able to share their experiences and have an equal say in the relationship.

If a man cannot accept that his partner is entitled to live her own life, then at least if she decides to leave he can try to respect her decision, however painful it may be, and not track her down or pump her family, friends or children to find out where she is in order to harass her, or exert more control over her life.

He should not succumb to the temptation to use the children: asking them to 'Tell Mummy I love her,' or saying, 'It was your mother's fault we aren't a family anymore.' He must accept that using children as a method of further control and abuse is destructive.

It may be hard, but the only course is to comply with the terms of protection orders and injunctions, and try to help himself by taking positive steps to understand the causes of the abuse and learn to deal with it in the future.

But on the positive side, it is not the end of the world. Even if the man must face the fact that there is no hope for the relationship, he may still be able to change his behaviour and begin a sharing relationship with someone else. Not only will his relationships with future partners be more fulfilling, but he will find it easier to cultivate real friendships and relate to other people in all spheres of his life.

### 'Stop using anger to control your partner'

An abusive man can learn that it is possible for anger to be kept in check. He must learn that it is not weak or unmanly to discuss things, express his emotions and vulnerability, rather than venting everything through anger, violence and abuse. In the meantime, he should consider his partner's safety. If he refuses to take steps to control his anger, he can choose to separate from his partner. He has a choice not to be violent.

I would like to say to any abusive man reading this: take a look at your behaviour. Try to recognise the ways in which you attempt to control your partner. Ask yourself: are you really angry because your shirt is not ironed, or is the real issue something deeper? Is it because she has somehow transgressed from the role you expect her to fulfil? Do you treat anyone else in this way, or is it only your partner?

Just because you got away with treating her in this way for a period of time does not mean you have to continue. You can begin to change the pattern by listing all the less obvious ways in which you might be trying to control your partner.

Do you interrupt her constantly? When she is asked a question, do you answer for her? Do you expect and demand more space than her in the home: like Guy, do you insist that your possessions or books are more important and therefore can be on show in the house, while hers are hidden away upstairs or in cupboards? Do you have your own office, den or workshop, while the only space she has for herself is the kitchen?

Do you ever bother to find out whether she wants to have sex every night, or is it just a masculine reflex action? You could try looking at sex differently, as a way of developing real closeness and trust. As something which is about love and tenderness, rather than the need to 'perform'.

Of course, there are going to be times when you differ greatly on something. But remember, a woman cannot be a mind reader: there is no point in losing your temper when she may not even know what is annoying you. Instead of exploding, 'You drive me mad!', why not start by saying, 'I think…', 'I feel…', 'I would like…' Approach things in a way that does not instantly imply blame and criticism.

Things are never black and white, right or wrong. People are different and are entitled to hold different views from yours. Instead of digging in and trying to prove a point all the time, why not say, 'Okay, that's your view, but what I feel is…'

One of the few men I have talked to who actually accepted responsibility for his behaviour and took positive steps to change was Lawrence, a bank clerk. He had been referred to a counselling group after the police had been called to his home because he had hit his wife. After two years with the group he admitted, 'The fact that I got arrested made me take a second look at what was happening. For too many years the general attitude has been that a man should be able to discipline his wife. That's stupid. The wife is a person, just like him.

'He has no right to discipline her any more than she has the right to discipline him. There are laws against this. There are laws against beating anyone, and too many times wife-beating is just seen as a domestic thing. Someone is being hurt, someone is being hurt badly, and the husband is getting away with it because it is a domestic thing. It isn't a domestic thing, it's an assault. No matter what you say about wife-beaters, in most cases he loves his wife and she loves him, but I don't know any of them who get violent with *other* people when they can't get their own way – only their wives.

'I think that somewhere in the back of my mind I thought home was my castle and I was the king. I think it's a case of thinking you are the boss, the big cheese, and people had better do as you say. That other guy, the guy I used to be, thought everyone else was at fault. He'd say, "They know I've got a bad temper, why do they push me?" But no one else is responsible for my temper, they can't make me do things. When I realised that, I thought, "Hey, there's something wrong here."

'I wouldn't go back to being the person I was under any conditions. I don't want anything to do with that person. I still get frustrated, but when things are at a point with my wife where it is so frustrating that you know if it goes on any further there is going to be a problem, I just simply say, "I can't handle this, I'm not in any position to handle this. I'll simply have to come back to this and walk away right now." That is the most important thing.

'We still have disagreements. I still get angry, but it's what you do with the anger. I'm a long way from being perfect, but I'm more perfect than I was two and a half years ago.'

The bottom line for an abusive man is: if he wants to find a way forward, he must accept that what he is really trying to do is control his partner. And that that is just not acceptable behaviour. He must understand that she has a right to her own opinions, that she is not simply an extension of himself, she is a human being in her own right, with a right to work and have friends and activities outside the relationship, if she desires. He has to recognise that he does not own her body, that she has a right to say no to sex and that he has no right to use force to make her submit.

He can learn to listen, rather than dictate, to be supportive, rather than critical, to discuss problems constructively, rather than resort to blame, name-calling or physical assault. His goal should be to develop a healthy respect for and empathy with all women, not just his partner.

Once he accepts all this, he can then learn how to act constructively, rather than destructively, in a relationship. He *can* unlearn what society has been teaching him for generations.

In conclusion, abusive men need to do the following:

- Stop denying that there is a problem.
- Accept responsibility for their behaviour.
- Know that whatever goes wrong in their relationship, men are not entitled to hit their partner or child.
- Remember that they are not alone; many men are conditioned to control women – but it is unacceptable. Domestic abuse and coercive control are against the law.
- Recognise how they have been abusing their power.
- Realise that they can change their abusive behaviour.
- Understand that abuse is learned behaviour rooted in sexist attitudes; what has been learned can be unlearned.
- Make a commitment to seek professional help.
- Recognise that women deserve to be treated as equals.

## For society

'What's the point of intervening? They'll only kiss and make up in the morning.' 'You spend all that time on paperwork and then they only drop the charges.' 'He just needs to cool off a bit – they'll be all lovey-dovey later. What's the point of arresting him?'

As already discussed, these sorts of negative attitudes are still common among the police – even after the publication of HMIC's ground-breaking reports – and they are also common among the public.

But there *is* a point to intervening, arresting and charging. And it is a major one: the single most important goal is to stop the abuse of women. One of the most potent ways of showing abusive men that what they are doing is wrong – rather than something which men are doing behind every door in the street, as one abuser put it – is to arrest and prosecute them.

It is not that the police do not want to help abused women; it is simply that, like the rest of society, they are frequently hoodwinked by myths. Often they do not recognise the seriousness of the problem until they actually see hideous injuries. What I would like to see is a strong police response. 'It's a one-off – I don't think we should do anything if he's only hit her once,' they say. But how do they know it is only once, when, as we have seen, both the men and the women deny and minimise what is happening? On average, a woman is assaulted 35 times before she calls the police for help.[83] And even if it has only happened once, I point out that there *will* be a next time. And next time she might be carried out on a stretcher.

'But you can't put the breadwinner in prison – you'll cause even more hardship by breaking up the family,' people say. I would answer that the family is already torn apart by violence. How does it help a woman if her partner is allowed to stay with her and possibly kill her next time, leaving the children without either parent if he is convicted of murder? Stopping him now will save everyone from years of misery. And if he is not stopped, it is likely that she will leave him anyway – so the family will still be broken up. Despite pressure to maintain the family unit, it must be recognised that a two-parent family is not the ideal when a child sees its mother being systematically battered and humiliated by its father.

'It's time-consuming and costly to get involved in "domestics"' is another objection I have heard. I would argue that, on the contrary, a strong police response acts as a deterrent and will actually save police time and money. If they do not arrest an abuser, they will usually find themselves being called out time and time again to the same house.

'But women don't want to see their men locked up' is another argument I hear frequently. It is hard to see the person you love locked up, but in the long term, it is the only way women will be protected. Even some of the men I speak to acknowledge this. They accept that without such harsh measures they would never have changed their ways.

Woman abuse is always treated differently from other crimes. If a woman was robbed in the street or her home was burgled, would the attitude be 'She wouldn't like to see the poor robber locked up'? In my view woman abuse should be seen as even more serious than other violent crimes, where strangers are involved, because the woman receives a double blow. Not only does she suffer the attack, but there is a terrible violation of trust – which is compounded by the fact that society does not really seem to care. And she lives with her attacker.

I do not like to see people thrown into prison any more than the next person. But it is dangerous to be sidetracked into saying things like 'He's as much a victim – it's not his fault, he's a product of a chauvinist society.' It is dangerous to say, 'He only needs counselling', because research shows that this simply does not act as a deterrent in the long term. If men commit other violent crimes, they are sent to prison, so why should it be any different if a man attacks a woman in the home? Without such deterrents, what is to stop men abusing women for generations to come?

As I have pointed out to many police officers over the years, arresting and charging is also important in that it educates people about the seriousness of the problem. Such a policy delivers four strong messages.

First, to the woman the message is that she is not to blame. She has not been a bad wife or mother. She is no different from someone who has been mugged or burgled. It shows her that she is important, that she deserves protection and that she *can* regain some real power to put an end to her suffering.

Second, to the abusive man the message is that what he is doing is *wrong,* that he has no justification for controlling women and that there is a price to pay.

Third, to society as a whole the message is that the abuse of women is unacceptable, criminal behaviour. Once that is universally recognised, police, healthcare professionals, neighbours, friends and family can feel that it is their right and duty to intervene when they suspect that a woman is being abused in the home.

The fourth message is to the next generation, to the children. They must be brought up knowing that violence towards women is not the norm but a punishable crime and that there are ways of handling problems other than being violent and abusive. Healthy relationships are based on equality and respect.

### 'Just calm down, mate'

The police do have the power to intervene when men abuse women in the home. The Police and Criminal Evidence Act of 1984 gives officers powers of arrest in cases where they have reasonable grounds to believe that an assault has taken place or may take place, however minor, or 'in order to protect a vulnerable person or child'. Guidance from national bodies like the Association of Chief Police Officers (ACPO) has reminded police officers of these powers.

HMIC showed that there is a huge inconsistency in rates of arrest for domestic violence between police forces. Its report for 2016 found that the arrest rate for domestic abuse perpetrators had fallen by 15 per cent. In some forces 75 per cent of domestic abuse perpetrators are not arrested.[84]

Still I hear of cases where, rather than arresting and charging, officers still say things like, 'Just calm down, mate,' or 'Don't worry, love, we've talked to him and he won't touch you now.' Little do they know that, once the police have left, many men resume hitting their partners. Getting a positive police response is often a postcode lottery. HMIC's initial report also found that in some forces, there are high levels of 'cautioning' as a way of dealing with abusive men, instead of charging them.[85] Cautioning is traditionally used for incidents which are considered 'slight' or are first-time offences.

But cautioning is not enough. For a start, it often leaves the woman exposed to an abuser who is likely to be even more irate because the police have been called. Imagine the burden that places on a woman who may already be terrified and confused by her partner's behaviour. If he is violent again, she has to make yet another call – and this time she is more aware of the consequences of that call. The pressures on her are doubled. She is also left in a vulnerable position, and may even become a murder statistic.

Also, as we have seen, Charm Syndrome Man is rarely abusive every day. He may be perfectly capable of behaving charmingly for months or more, but he will resume the cycle of violence some time or other.

And women whose partners have indeed been 'good boys' during the cautioning period and have then reverted to violent behaviour will be reluctant to call the police a second time. After all, what good did it do the first time?

Cautioning does not deliver a strong enough message that an abusive man's behaviour is unacceptable. Cautioning puts the crime on the same level as juvenile crime and shoplifting by elderly people (the main areas in which officers caution rather than arrest). It is time to stop delaying real progress by advocating such futile measures. In my experience, unless the cycle of violence is stopped as early as possible, it will only escalate – no matter how many cautions are issued.

Charging, not cautioning, *must* be the norm – no more of the 'Just calm down, mate' attitude which results in abusers, such as Hazel's husband, being taken around the corner to the local pub by the police, rather than to the police station.

## 'We understand what you're going through'

Since a police officer is often the first person a woman encounters when she cries for help, the police need specific training in how to handle and understand the complex power dynamics of woman abuse. It is imperative that they take abused women seriously, and avoid implying blame by asking questions such as 'What did you do to make him hit you?'

HMIC's report found a number of weaknesses with police training. For example, training is often delivered through e-learning packages, which means that officers sit at a computer, clicking through questions rather than engaging face to face with an expert. With the latter, they would have the opportunity to ask questions and get to grips with difficult issues, and any negative attitudes or opinions they expressed would be openly challenged. HMIC also recommended that training should not just be a 'one-off', but should be given to officers at regular intervals, to refresh their knowledge and skills.

Without specialist training, officers will not be able to spot the complex risks and dynamics of domestic violence. The police now have tools for risk assessment, which – when used correctly – enable them to identify risk, and refer women to the right kind of support. Risk assessment is a blunt instrument, though – women can rarely be cleanly divided into 'standard', 'medium' or 'high' risk, because risk factors are constantly changing. Police officers must use any risk-assessment tools in combination with their well-informed professional opinion; that is why training, and working closely with experts like Refuge, is so important.

Progress *is* being made. The Home Secretary now monitors the police response to domestic violence, and the College of Policing is developing a national training for police officers. They are even devising professional standards to make police officers responding to abused women more accountable. Police forces now have special units to deal specifically with the problem of domestic violence. This is a positive thing, and when such units work, they work extremely well. It is good for women and agencies to know that there is a specialist officer who can be contacted.

A positive response is when the police come immediately, when they interview the parties separately, when they gather evidence, take statements, take photographs, use body-worn cameras,  check previous incidents, conduct risk assessments and develop safety plans. And when they arrest and charge. This is what will increase women's confidence in the police. It is vital that chief constables and senior officers show strong leadership on this issue in order to ensure an effective response to incidents of domestic violence.

The police have also become much better at liaising with other agencies – called a 'coordinated community response' – to ensure that women do not fall through the gaps. Multi-agency risk-assessment conferences (MARACs) are now commonplace across the country. MARACs are a forum of professionals drawn from local agencies, including police, social services, health, education, probation and domestic violence services. They allow everyone involved in a case to get together and make plans to ensure the safety of women at the risk of death or serious harm.

### 'We will prosecute'

There is considerable legislation, together with several civil remedies, which in theory afford abused women protection.

The Police and Criminal Evidence Act 1984, the Criminal Justice Act 1988, Offences Against the Person Act 1861, Sexual Offences Act 1956, Public Order Act 1986 and Criminal Damage Act 1971 all relate in varying degrees either to offences that can be carried out against women or to the police and court powers to deal with those offences.

The Protection from Harassment Act of 1997 prohibited a person from pursuing any course of conduct which amounts to harassment of another, which he knows or ought to know amounts to harassment of the other. Under the Harassment Act it is an offence to put another in fear of violence and the court can impose a restraining order on the offender for an indefinite period of time, which if breached, can result in imprisonment of up to five years. An injunction can be granted and breach of that injunction, without a reasonable excuse, is an arrestable offence and damages may be awarded for any anxiety or financial loss caused by the harassment. In 2012, the Protection from Harassment Act was amended to introduce two new specific criminal offences: 'stalking' and 'stalking involving fear of violence or serious alarm and distress'. In 1996, Part IV of the Family Law Act created non-molestation orders and occupation orders designed to protect abused women further.

In 2004, the Domestic Violence, Crime and Victims Act, as well as extending the availability of restraining orders to all offences, provided the court with the power to make a restraining order even when a person has been acquitted, where the court considers it necessary to do so to protect a person from ongoing stalking or harassment from the defendant. Since 2014, women have also benefited from Domestic Violence Protection Orders (DVPOs), whereby a perpetrator can be banned with immediate effect from returning to a residence and from having contact with the victim for up to 28 days, allowing a woman time to consider her options and get the support she needs. Sentencing guidelines also clearly state that domestic violence can be seen as an 'aggravating factor' and thus increase the penalty for offences.

The most recent change in legislation came in 2015, when the Serious Crime Act created a new offence of controlling or coercive behaviour in an intimate or family relationship. I am ambivalent about this new law. As you can see from the list above, we already have enough laws to protect women – the problem is that they are not implemented properly. The police don't even arrest when there is evidence of serious physical violence, so how are police and juries ever going to understand complex concepts like coercive control?

Controlling behaviour can be incredibly subtle and isn't always 'coercive'. Extreme jealousy and possessiveness, for example, can be dressed up to look like 'care' or 'concern'. Providing evidence of such behaviours to satisfy criminal standards is likely to be extremely difficult. In the months since the law was introduced, this has been borne out – in the summer of 2016, the law firm Simpson Millar submitted a Freedom of Information request which found that of those who answered, most forces had launched fewer than five coercive control actions between December 2015 and June 2016, with several having charged nobody with the offence.[86] The new law could also have unintended consequences – it could lead to police officers treating it as a separate, less serious category of crime; also, serious physical offences could be downgraded and perpetrators undercharged.

In February 2017, Prime Minister Theresa May launched a major consultation across government to result in a domestic violence and abuse act, consolidating relevant legislation and introducing new measures to help victims. This has the potential to bring the sea change needed to give women the protection they deserve; but at the time of writing, those who work supporting survivors are still waiting to hear more detail.

The Crown Prosecution Service has made strides in recent years when it comes to domestic violence. It has increased the number of prosecutions and improved training, and senior staff have shown real leadership. However, historically – like society as a whole – the Crown Prosecution Service has been guilty of treating woman abuse as a less serious crime than other forms of violence.

All too often, cases are downgraded. Sentencing, too, must be appropriate to the crime. Violent men are constantly being let off with suspended sentences, probation orders and short-term sentences. Sentences should be as stiff as those imposed for any other violent crime, not only in cases of domestic violence, but also where a woman is sexually abused by her partner. And that means recognising that rape is as much a crime when the woman lives with her aggressor as when she is attacked by a total stranger. In fact, I would like to suggest that we go one step further and pass a gender-specific law which states that 'woman abuse' is a crime which warrants appropriate sentencing.

Men and women must not be persuaded to attend mediation and conciliation sessions; courts must take rigorous action when injunctions are breached. If abusers breach conditions of bail, they should not be allowed bail a second time. If we really want to find a way forward to a time when men no longer abuse women, then the police, the Crown Prosecution Service and the judiciary must work together and take positive steps to prevent it. They must show society that woman abuse is a crime and as such will not be tolerated.

In short, if we want to see real change, we must address the whole response of the criminal justice system in cases of domestic violence:

- Improved police response is required, including strengthened pro-arrest or mandatory arrest policies, improved collection of evidence and an end to the routine release of the offender on bail.
- Abusers must be held to account. There should be stronger sanctions against abusers, an end to the routine downgrading of charges and more rigorous enforcement of criminal and civil legislation. Overall, we need to see use of interventions that have been proven to be most effective in stopping abusive men from re-offending. This means not imposing fines or sending violent men on perpetrator programmes (the flaws of which are discussed opposite) but instead using custodial sentences to fit the crime and ensuring there are consequences when civil remedies – like non-molestation orders – are breached.
- Comprehensive training in domestic violence should be provided for all legal practitioners at every level.
- Greater protection and support for women in courts is required. Special measures – a screen so that a witness doesn't have to see her perpetrator, for example – should be standard practice when a woman is testifying against her abuser.
- The family courts should ensure no woman is questioned by her perpetrator, and end the presumption that contact with both parents is preferable. Children must be protected from unsafe contact with their fathers.

- When it comes to cases of domestic violence, the criminal and civil courts must be joined up and ensure they are sharing information.

## 'Shouldn't we counsel the men?'

Many people consider that the way forward is to set up programmes to counsel abusive men. When I tell people that arresting and charging can deter the abuse of women, they argue that the way to deal with abusive men is through men's programmes (or perpetrator programmes, as they are often called).

I am seriously concerned about the current trend for perpetrator programmes. As part of the solution to domestic violence, the theory goes that we should be encouraging abusers to change their behaviour. Of course, in an ideal world this would be true. As I have already said, I do believe that abusers can change their behaviour – but first they must recognise it and take responsibility. Yet there is no evidence that perpetrator programmes work. The largest study to date on the effectiveness of perpetrator programmes, Project Mirabal, published in 2015, found that after 12 months of sessions, 23 per cent of men still punched or kicked furniture and walls, slammed doors or smashed things, and 10 per cent still made threats to kill.[87] Yes, the number of men still physically abusing their partners reduced (although not to zero, it must be said) – but 41 per cent of women said their perpetrator still did things that made them feel scared and 75 per cent said they still felt they would have to be very careful around him if he was in a bad mood.[88] These figures do represent a reduction in these behaviours over the 12-month period, but unacceptable levels of abuse remain – and how long will these reductions last, particularly when men go back into an unchanged, sexist society? What is more, the positive outcomes for children in the Mirabal study were minimal. The number of mothers who said they felt worried about leaving their children alone with the perpetrator remained unchanged; as did the number of mothers reporting that their children were nervous or clingy.[89]

This is psychological abuse: a kind of mental torture which keeps the woman on edge, never knowing when her partner's threats and insinuations are for real. The evidence on perpetrator programmes is clear and many women are still left walking on egg shells, living in fear. Unless this changes, how can spending money on such programmes be justified, when we do not have enough services for women fleeing violence? Anything less than a total end to all forms of abuse and controlling behaviour cannot be seen as success.

Understandably, women hope that perpetrator programmes will change their partner. Women have made huge emotional investments in their relationships. They have tried everything to make it work, including adapting their behaviour to meet their partner's demands. They don't want their children to be fatherless, or for their partners to go to prison. They live in hope that their partners will change. Perpetrator programmes can appear like the last beacon of hope. But abusers can only change if they accept responsibility for their violent behaviour.

Tellingly, Mirabal finds that after 12 months, 71 per cent of perpetrators still attempted to justify or make excuses for their behaviour (down from 91 per cent). Sixty-one per cent of women said that the perpetrator blamed her for his abusive behaviour (down from 84 per cent).[90] For the majority of men, the pattern is unchanged. In keeping with the abuser's modus operandi, he is never wrong. I would prefer to see money spent on training all professionals – not only the police, but doctors, social workers and counsellors – to respond appropriately to the men as well as to the women. However, there is a more immediate priority and that is to pour all available resources into helping the thousands of women and children who are suffering, and into educating society and eliminating gender inequality, rather than concentrating on counselling individual men.

In an ideal world, once we have established and implemented an arrest-and-charge policy, challenged society's traditional attitudes, provided immediate help and resources for abused women and their children, and made more people aware of the extent of the problem, then (and only then) can we begin to look at men's programmes – not as the sole answer but in conjunction with sentencing.

### 'What's in a name?'

Before we can even attempt to solve the problem of woman abuse, we first have to recognise it. And that begins with the very language we use to describe it. The issue is not 'domestic violence', 'conjugal violence' or 'abusive relationships'. All those terms imply mutual abuse, and in doing so share the blame between the man and the woman.

Our government's own definition of domestic violence does not even mention men and women. It simply says that domestic violence is any incident or pattern of abuse 'between those aged 16 or over who are, or have been, intimate partners or family members regardless of gender or sexuality'.[91] This overlooks the fact that domestic violence is a deeply gendered crime.

As I have already said, the way you describe a problem affects how you see it and what you do about it. What we are talking about is 'woman abuse'. The abuse of women is about behaviour which is designed to control and subjugate a woman, through physical, psychological, emotional and verbal abuse, aimed at inspiring fear, humiliation, shame and guilt. The very first step society has to take is to stop skirting around the issue with wishy-washy terminology. What we are talking about is 'woman abuse', and something must be done about it. We need definitions and laws which see woman abuse for what it really is – male violence and control of women on a huge scale – so that we can implement the right solutions and ultimately save lives.

### 'Her needs are special'

Doctors, nurses in casualty units, members of the clergy, social workers and other professionals should be encouraged to report abuse, keep accurate records so that the extent of the abuse can be monitored, and help to educate the public by using posters and so on. Like the police, most agencies have got better at this – for example, midwives are encouraged to routinely ask pregnant women if they are being abused. Professionals now have a better understanding of the need to coordinate their response.

Yet they are not always following through. The Home Office's own analysis has shown that in 76 per cent of domestic homicide reviews – undertaken when a woman is killed, so that agencies can understand what lessons can be learned – communication and information-sharing between agencies was identified as an issue.[92] Eighty-five per cent recorded record-keeping as an issue. This is a tragedy. Just think of the lives that could be saved if only agencies could get this relatively simple thing right.

In 73 per cent of the domestic homicide reviews sampled, victims or perpetrators presented to agencies with possible signs of domestic abuse, but this was not recognised or explored further. Very often, medical professionals – doctors, midwives, health visitors – are best placed to notice something is wrong. They may be the first person to whom a woman discloses her abuse. They must *all* be trained to spot domestic violence, so that when women come to them complaining of stress, depression, dependency on drugs or alcohol, they can ask the right questions in order to discover whether there is something more concealed behind these symptoms. It may simply be a case of asking some basic questions as a matter of routine, such as 'Does your partner hit you?' or 'Are you happy with your partner?' or 'Are you frightened of him?'

Such professionals need to consider their actions when dealing with these cases. In the same way that it would be inappropriate for a police officer to question a woman in the same room as her abuser, a woman should not be examined in front of her abuser. How can she speak freely and without fear when the man who is making her life hell and terrifying her with threats is in the same room? The way a woman is treated from the moment she first asks for help is of vital importance. Her situation must be treated seriously, and her needs should be addressed immediately, no matter how busy the doctor, social worker or counsellor may be. It may have taken that woman months, perhaps years, to reach the point of picking up a phone and asking for help. If at that point the person she turns to is unsympathetic, however unintentionally, she may never seek help again. She may even end up as a murder statistic.

First and foremost, the woman must feel safe. When she calls out for help she is often in fear for her life and for the lives of her children. In the eyes of her abuser she has committed the ultimate sin of abandonment. He may have treated her with utter contempt during the relationship, but the last thing he wants is to be deserted, because that damages his ability to be in control. The symbiotic bond between himself and his partner has been severed, the woman he has depended upon to make him feel a real man has left him. In this state he is usually very desperate, and frequently very dangerous.

It is at this point that a woman needs protection most. Her partner will try everything from threatening suicide to vowing to kill the woman or her children. Such threats must always be taken seriously, since in most cases these men have already proved just how violent they can be, and the reality is that many women are tracked down by their partners and physically attacked after they have left home.

However, many men use more subtle appeals: an abuser may try to charm the woman with professions of love and remorse, he will beg forgiveness and promise to change – if only she will come back to him. He may bombard her with letters or flowers. It should never be forgotten that a woman may still have very strong feelings towards her partner. However much she has suffered, it is rarely possible for her to be single-minded about leaving.

She will be torn by feelings of love, pity and guilt at breaking up her family, and in this emotional maelstrom it is all too easy for her partner to remind her of the charming, loving, caring side of his character, the side which she fell in love with and which she wants to return for good. It is all too easy for her to push the bad times out of her mind and to believe that he will change. The professional needs to be very aware of this heightened vulnerability when a woman first leaves her abuser and, if necessary, to take steps to help her find out about her legal rights.

However, if the woman does return to her abuser, even if she does so time and time again, it is important to understand the dilemmas she faces, rather than blame her for going back. However much an adviser may disagree with her choices and decisions, they must still be respected.

In order to protect the woman as much as is humanly possible, confidentiality is vital, especially if a woman has not actually left her partner but is seeking advice on whether to do so. If her partner should discover that she has told anyone about her situation, she may be in more danger than ever.

What is also vital is that abused women should receive the right *sort* of help. Something as seemingly minor as the way a question is constructed can make all the difference to a woman. For example, if a professional looks at a woman's black eye and asks, 'Have you been fighting with your partner?', he or she is implying that the woman is, partly at least, to blame.

Remember that when women ask for help they are invariably ashamed, humiliated, frightened and prone to blaming themselves, since that is what their abusers have done. In this state, even the slightest hint that a doctor, counsellor or social worker is in any way sceptical about a woman's story, or feels she is in some way responsible for her situation, can drive that woman to desperation.

The woman already feels isolated and alone, she feels that no one will listen, believe her or even care. Her fears need to be dispelled, and she needs the reassurance that she is not alone, that many, many other women have gone through similar experiences, that what has happened to her is no reflection on her, and that, above all, it is not her fault. No woman should be held accountable for the behaviour of an abusive man.

If counsellors and other professionals believe any of the myths about the causes of woman abuse, such as that it happens because the women have masochistic tendencies, then, even though in the short term they may be able to offer women assistance, in the long term they will actually help to perpetuate the abuse by cloaking the real issue with excuses.

Abused women must be helped to understand that their abusers act the way they do, not because the women are bad or inadequate people, not because the women attract violence, and not because the men have had one drink too many, but because such men believe they have the right to control and subjugate them, a belief which is encouraged and reinforced by society.

Counsellors and other professionals also need to be aware that abused women are survivors and that, because of that, they will have adopted techniques of coping, such as minimising or denying the abuse. Like the hostages in the Stockholm bank they may have learned to survive by adapting their behaviour to avoid situations which may spark off the abuse. All these tactics are vital to their safety and sanity while they are living with their abusers, yet once they have made the break, once they are out of danger, it is time for them to vent all the anger and hurt they have suppressed for so long.

Because they are so used to minimising their pain and excusing their partners' behaviour, no one should be surprised if women gloss over certain events, if they hold back details or if, having firmly blanked out events which are particularly painful, they cannot at first recall them. Some women seem to have so little to say at first that professionals may even wonder why they are seeking help. It may be a long time before they can admit the full extent of the abuse, but they need to be encouraged to talk through even their most traumatic memories, before the process of rebuilding their confidence and self-esteem can begin. They need to be shown that the survival techniques they adopted, often unconsciously, were right at the time, but now that they are free, and safe, they can begin to be assertive and independent again.

Even when women move on, it is important for them to keep in contact with the professionals, if possible, so that they know that they are only a telephone call away from advice and support in the future.

## 'Take it from the top'

The Government should be funding more national campaigns to educate not only professionals, but the general public. We need to teach children about woman abuse, healthy relationships, equality and respect, and that violence is not the way to deal with problems.

In 2017, the Government announced that Relationships and Sex Education (RSE) would be made statutory in schools. This is a good first step towards a better and safer future for young people, but RSE needs to deliver the right things – education around consent, healthy relationships and different forms of abuse, but also an understanding that gender inequality lies at the root of violence against women – in order to be effective.

We need to train teachers to look for tell-tale indicators in the children. If they have poor concentration, are often tired, their performance is not what it should be, they act out, get into fights or are involved in bullying, or seem withdrawn, depressed, jumpy or anxious, or alternatively, if they are always the peacemaker, or afraid to fail, it could be that they are living in a violent home. Schools need to develop comprehensive programmes to help them recognise and respond to such abuse. They may also be able to help the women.

Women must be made aware of their rights: leaflets could be inserted into information packs given out by midwives after giving birth, and posters and literature could be placed in nurseries, doctors' surgeries, clinics and social services departments.

We also need more TV and radio campaigns telling people that woman abuse is a crime against society and showing women how they can spot the signs.

In addition to refuges, the government also needs to provide adequate funding for the range of other specialist services that support women and children to escape abuse and rebuild their lives, such as Independent Domestic Violence Advocates (IDVAs), community-based programmes and specialist services for black, Asian and minority ethnic women. It needs to provide nursery places to enable women who want to leave abusive men to go back to work. It needs to give them better educational opportunities and to establish job-retraining programmes.

People ask, 'Why should the Government have to do this?' My answer is that woman abuse is a serious social problem. It means that there are many women who are unable to fulfil their potential and contribute to society because of that abuse. It is estimated that domestic violence costs England and Wales £16 billion a year, including lost economic output, costs to public services and the human and emotional cost.[93]

Refuge's specialist services save the health service and criminal justice system £5.9 million a year. Funding domestic violence services and addressing domestic violence through the means listed above make economic sense, because eliminating woman abuse would mean fewer women on income support, fewer children in children's homes or in care, less demand on police time and resources, and less demand on housing and social services.

### 'How can I help?'

Neighbours and friends need to know that they can – and should – help if they suspect that someone close to them is being abused. In cases of actual violence the answer is always to call the police. Nobody is suggesting you should stand between a man with a hatchet in his hand, and his partner.

Many people, quite understandably, worry about interfering, but it should be remembered that many female homicide victims are killed by present or former male partners. A phone call to the police could save a woman's life.

It may be that a friend or neighbour can keep an eye on the situation, and wait for the right moment to approach the woman and reassure her that she has friends who are willing to help, that she has a lifeline should she require it. An abused woman often feels so isolated and alone that just knowing there is someone out there who cares about her, and does not blame her, may be the spur she needs to seek help.

However, it is important to be patient, to listen, and not to force her to take decisions until she is ready. It may be hard for an outsider to understand, but an abused woman is rarely able to walk away from her abuser without conquering fears and feelings of guilt which at times seem insurmountable. It does not help her to have someone constantly telling her that she should leave without a second thought. A well-meaning friend who criticises her for staying, tells her she is crazy, will only intensify her confusion, guilt and lack of self-esteem.

Running down her partner does not help either, as the woman may leap to his defence, or feel that there is something wrong with her for having chosen the wrong man. ('He is so bad; I chose him; so I must be bad too.') Instead, the most important thing to do is to assure the woman that she is not to blame, that she is not responsible for her abuser's behaviour. It is necessary to bolster her self-confidence and courage by giving her the credit for coping so well, to emphasise her strength, show her that she will be able to survive without her partner, and make her aware of agencies she can turn to for help, if and when she feels ready to leave.

If friends and family need information on how to help people close to them, staff at organisations such as Refuge are always ready to offer advice. Refuge also runs a website called **www.1in4women.com**, which provides lots of information on how friends and family can support loved ones who may be experiencing domestic violence.

## 'Women are just as important'

Arrest and prosecution is the most palpable signal now and to future generations that woman abuse should be stamped out, but it is not enough. Nor is it enough just to dot the country with refuges. If we are ever going to see any real progress, the root cause of the problem must also be addressed. If abusers are to cease the kind of controlling behaviour which they believe to be their right, society has to remove that sense of right, and in order to do so it must take a long hard look at the attitudes towards men and women and their roles which society fosters. And it must make some fundamental changes.

As long as women are made to feel inferior to men; as long as they have less representation in the higher echelons of power; as long as they have less access to highly paid jobs; and as long as they are taught that their sense of worth depends on finding and keeping a man, they will always be targets for abusive men.

This is particularly important in ending the emotional and verbal abuse of women, since punishment for such behaviour is infinitely harder to secure than if a woman has broken bones to show for her pain. In many cases of emotional and verbal abuse even the woman does not realise that she has any right to complain, or that coercive control is against the law. She may not even be aware that she is abused. She only knows that she is unhappy, and that she feels manipulated and dominated to a suffocating degree.

We need to encourage equality of the sexes, rather than resting on our laurels and pretending that discrimination against women is a thing of the past. We must challenge the traditional idea, which still prevails, that men wield the power and women are subservient. It is this idea that acts as a springboard for the abuse of women. Since we learn it almost from the cradle – by listening to our parents and teachers and observing their behaviour, through children's literature, songs and television, even through the clothes we are dressed in and the toys we are given – we have to begin the re-education process early on.

If we teach children that they are equals, they are more likely to act that way as adults. We should teach little boys that girls deserve respect, that they are not just 'sissies', that they are just as important as men, and that above all boys do not have the right to dominate girls. They must not grow up to be controllers.

We can also teach children about anger – that it is not something uncontrollable, something which cannot be helped, but a simple emotion which tells us when something in our life feels wrong. How we respond to feelings of anger is a choice, but learning to pause, take a breath and think about what underpins the anger takes practice. Children can be taught that it is possible to be assertive and recognise and express their thoughts and feelings without resorting to aggression or violence.

In later life, boys who grow up learning that women have a right to their own opinions will be able to express their own without resorting to abuse, and see that it is better to calmly negotiate differences rather than use physical or verbal aggression. If, from an early age, boys and girls are taught that men have no right to be violent, women may be better equipped in later life, should they find themselves living with an abusive man. Ultimately, they may find it easier to leave.

Children learn from their parents. Although, as I have mentioned, this is not the cause of woman abuse, when they see their fathers beat their mothers, or they are hit themselves, they receive the message that love and violence somehow go together, that it is okay to use physical and verbal violence to get what you want, that it is okay to try to control other people.

Both boys and girls must be taught that love and abuse do not have to go hand in hand; parents should never smack their children, because this sends the message that it is okay to hit the people you love. Boys, in particular, are already surrounded by messages which tell them to be aggressive, so being hit themselves only strengthens the idea that violence is an acceptable way of getting what they want.

However, it is pointless to try to show children – especially boys – that violence is wrong, if all around them they see it on the television and in the cinema, and glorified in cartoons and books.

Nor is it any good if they constantly see women being pictured in degrading poses in pornographic magazines, pop videos and films, or being shown washing clothes and cooking meals in adverts.

Of course, not all women want to pursue careers. The important thing is that women should have a choice about the way they live their lives. And men should also be able to stay at home with the children, without being ridiculed. Millions of women enjoy being housewives and mothers, and have no desire to do anything else, but the important issue is that they should devote themselves to being wives and mothers because that is what they want to do, rather than unquestioningly taking on a role for which they feel their families and society have groomed them.

Choice is what it is all about, and from an early age children of both sexes should be brought up to respect the fact that women – and men – have many choices about the way they live their lives. They do not have to be bound by a tradition which says men control and women obey.

We need to educate our society through the media, through plays, TV soap operas, books and magazines. This has begun to happen: unlike when I first wrote this book, magazine editors and television executives are happy to produce stories on domestic violence and even feminism. But we need more media stories that reflect the full range of women's experiences, including psychological abuse, controlling behaviour and financial abuse, as well as other forms of gender violence like so-called 'honour'-based violence, forced marriage and FGM.

We should discourage pornography and advertising which shows women in a negative light. We could do with some enlightened storylines in children's books. For example, mothers – whether humans, rabbits, bears or pigs – could occasionally be seen doing more taxing things than making sandwiches and beds. Perhaps Daddy Pig could make the dinner for a change. And in adventure stories perhaps little girls could have some intrepid adventures, while little boys could sometimes be depicted as having gentle, compassionate sides to their character.

Curricula in school should be balanced, so that girls are not discouraged from studying traditionally 'masculine' subjects such as sciences or engineering.

When these girls grow up, if they decide to have children, we could help them to make choices by providing decent childcare, better training and better employment opportunities to help them return to work if they wish.

Many women find it difficult to leave their abusive partners not just because they are emotionally dependent on them, but because they are also financially dependent. Providing better and higher-paid employment for women and affordable housing prospects would also help to increase a woman's sense of her own worth, and the idea of leaving her abuser would become less daunting. And in addition to boosting a woman's self-esteem, such resources help redress the balance of power and encourage women to break the pattern of abusive control. Woman abuse is not an individual problem, it is a *social* problem that requires structural and institutional changes if we want to see the current harrowing statistics decrease.

The way forward for society is to aim at three goals: protection, provision and prevention. The main objective is to make abusive men accountable for their actions, but in the short term the priority is to provide refuges and community-based specialist services where women can feel safe and welcomed and can benefit from sound medical, legal and financial advice. In the long term, the ultimate goal is to alter society's view, through education, that men are entitled to control women.

## Life after Charm Syndrome Man

I began this book with the story of Melinda, who was 'devastated' by her husband Trevor's charm when they first met. Eleven months later, he hit her for the first time. Finally, after 12 years of marriage, and three years of trying to make the break, she left him for good.

Hers – like those of all our six women – is an encouraging story. She left her job in the city and, with a loan, set up a small business which flourished so well she was able to buy her own house. 'I can't tell you the joy of that house being *mine*,' she told me. 'I know I can go home, shut the door and not be afraid of anything. I can switch on the TV when I want, the children and I can eat when we want and what we want. We can go out when we like. It is such a liberating feeling, it is impossible to explain to someone who has never gone through what I did with Trevor.

'Then, about six months ago, I met a man who I've fallen completely in love with, and he feels the same way. He's great with the kids and they've come to accept him,' she told me. 'He showed me what normal life should be – because I had forgotten what normal life was. I feel so loved and cherished by him. He treats me with respect – it is wonderful. He isn't at all violent. But the important thing is that I don't feel I *need* him to be happy. Having that time to myself has shown me that just being free and in control of my life is enough. This man is just the icing on the cake.

'I had always had the idea that what happened with Trevor never could or would happen to me. I would never be abused by a man. And I was. But that doesn't mean to say it is going to happen again, or that I was attracted to it, or that it was my fault. That awareness that it is something which could happen to anybody has helped me over and over again.'

Hazel has brought up her two children on her own, and her self-esteem and confidence have grown enormously over the years. When she left Jimmy, she felt physically bruised, psychologically scarred and sexually humiliated: 'I felt that nobody would ever want me after what he had put me through. I felt drained, just drained. As if I was nothing, worthless. The sexual abuse was the worst. It got to a stage where I couldn't imagine enjoying love-making. Sexual abuse is a horrible cruel thing to do to anyone. It stunts you emotionally.'

A few months later, she told me: 'At one stage I could only sit in women's company. Now I can be with men, but I'm always on my guard. Because of the way I feel, nothing can develop, and I feel threatened if somebody starts to like me too much. I'm all right as long as there is no involvement.'

However, when I last saw her, she was much stronger. 'The thing to do is to think really clearly and *don't* think that it is your fault and blame yourself,' she said. 'It *is* difficult. Even now I've still got problems to sort out, but it's worth it. I've now got my confidence back, and I really feel as if I'm getting my life together now. My children are so happy, I know I've done the right thing.

'Once you're through, there's no looking back. I know I'll never be abused again. It's wonderful to feel that I'm clean, that this is *my* body, and I'm in charge of my body. If I make a mistake now, it's *my* mistake, and anything I do in life is *mine*. I appreciate different things now. And I like *me*. For a long time I didn't like me. For a long time there was nothing about me I could like. When you're abused for so long, there's nothing left for you to like.

'Now I realise I didn't deserve to be treated like that. Nobody does. There are certain times when the fear comes back, but I can control it now. Once you come through it, you're a stronger person. Life is just so good. Even if I was only given a year to live, I'd rather be the way I am now than the way I was. The days are lovely, life is so lovely...'

Rebecca, as I mentioned earlier, decided to stay with Ralph – at least until the children were older – but she took an enjoyable part-time job at a local art gallery. Ralph made an enormous fuss to begin with, but she held her ground. 'He hasn't changed at all, he is still as domineering as ever,' she told me, 'but I have changed. That is the difference. I feel much stronger. When he criticises me and gets angry I still get upset, but somewhere inside a little voice pipes up, "Remember it's his problem, not yours", and I cope.

'At the back of my mind I always know that when the children are older I *can* leave. It's as if I have a compartment in my head devoted to thinking about that day. I imagine doing absolutely everything that I want to do. It helps to get me through the grim days.'

Sally re-married (happily this time) and raised a family. She told me: 'For a long time I didn't trust men. But Graham has great sympathy with women. There is no question of him being controlling, or dominating me. We talk about everything. He supports my work – in fact I think he even puts *my* work above his sometimes, which takes some getting used to after the way Guy behaved!

'I think it is very important for women to know that the bad times pass. You *do* feel panicky – I did. I thought I couldn't live without Guy. I thought I would never get over it. The temptation to go back to what was familiar was very, very strong. But no one knows what is around the corner – for me there was a new job and, eventually, Graham. You do survive and you do recover. That feeling of being lost does go away. And you get a tremendous sense of freedom instead.

'I remember one day I suddenly thought to myself, "I can do exactly what I please today. I don't have to wonder what Guy will say if he walks through the door. I don't have to worry what sort of mood he'll be in. I don't have to keep looking over my shoulder." And instead of panicking, I felt so *free*. I got out all the books I wanted to read, which he had never let me display in the living room, and I found all the records he wouldn't let me play in case they damaged his damn stylus, and it felt so wonderful. I got an almost childish pleasure out of it.

'Even if I hadn't met Graham, I know that I was happier without Guy than with him. Of course, there were good times with Guy, but the bad outweighed the good ten times over.'

Beverley got together with a new boyfriend, Mark. She told me: 'When I was with Dave I could never just be me and express how I felt. I was always very careful what I said, in case I incurred his anger and abuse. I would always censor my behaviour. I was always looking over my shoulder. Now I don't have to do that. I don't feel that Mark likes just a part of me that suits him. Or a part of me that is going to behave in a way that won't incur anger or criticism. I feel valued. All of me. I feel accepted.

'A good relationship is one which doesn't take anything away from you. It leaves you a whole person, but in a connection with someone else, which can make you more of a person. Mark is lovely. Very easy-going. Sometimes I have a little panic,' she laughs. 'I feel this is too good to be true. I almost want to run away, in case it goes wrong!

'When I met Dave I thought I'd chosen the right man, so I keep asking myself, "How do you know now?" But Mark isn't jealous or possessive. There *are* a lot of similarities about the way I felt about Dave, but Dave was obsessive, controlling, whereas Mark is gentle, happy with his life. He's not dependent on me. I do worry, but my instincts tell me it is different this time.

'And you know the most amazing thing? Feeling safe in bed! Going to bed with Mark is so lovely because I feel *safe*. When you are in bed with someone you are at your most loving, but you are also at your most vulnerable. With Dave that was when I felt at my most unsafe. I never knew whether I was going to be loved or hurt. If I was awake, I'd always have to face sex, yet he was impotent, but for years I was never allowed to say that word. I used to think I'd love to creep up on him while he was having breakfast and yell it!

'Finally I'm accepting that it is okay to be *safe* with someone in bed. That it is inconceivable that anyone should be angry and violent and hurtful. It is a revelation. It is wonderful. On one occasion I just welled up and cried and cried. I told Mark how I felt and he was so surprised.

'He's listened an awful lot. A lot of people would say, "How could you stand it? Why didn't you leave him before?" Or, "Well, what must Dave have been going through?" Mark hasn't said any of that. In fact one of the first things he said to me was, "You're not responsible for his behaviour." I was really surprised at that! Because that's the most important thing to believe. Mark has never done any macho stuff and said, "What a horrible person", but he's told me on several occasions that it wasn't my fault.'

Laura moved in with Peter, who had been a friend of hers for many years. 'Peter didn't know about the physical abuse, but he was aware of the way James spoke to me, and he knew he was having an affair with somebody else, and he felt that I was getting a raw deal, although he never said anything at the time,' she recalls.

'Gradually we got close. But there have been terribly violent scenes with James. He was capable of driving up and down the street and waiting behind a parked car until Peter came back, then he'd set upon him and attack him. I felt terrible, because I had an injunction which protected me. James wasn't allowed to come to the house or intimidate me, or harass me in any way, but what he'd done was attack Peter in front of me. I felt as if he was taking the violence that I had had, instead of me – so we ended up going back to court again, and they said that the injunction covered harassing Peter too. But it hasn't stopped the threatening phone calls. He still phones up and threatens to kill me. It terrifies me. It has worn us down a lot. In James's eyes I had committed the ultimate in disobedience, if you like – I mean, if he saw our life together as trying to get me under control, I'd finally escaped and I was out of control.'

Of her relationship with Peter, she told me: 'After putting up with so much, and finally making the break, I'm never going to put up with abuse again. Because of that I'm desperately untrusting of Peter, and I know that I've pushed him deliberately. I mean, not kind of consciously, but I know I was seeing how far I could go at times. I was saying, "Is this real or is he going to hit me if I carry on like this?" I suppose I had to test him, because I couldn't believe it wasn't going to happen to me again.

'I still can't believe that I am with a man who is gentle and sweet, and everything else. Peter couldn't be more loving, and we couldn't have a more wonderful love life, but I still can't be sure. I just don't know...

'I gather that James's relationship with the woman he went off with has ended in some kind of violent situation, which actually reassures me,' she says, apologetically. 'I mean, I'm sorry, but it does. It's a slight case of my rubbing my hands and saying, "Well, it wasn't all my fault. I didn't bring it on myself." Because I remember this girl saying to people that James was the most gentle man she'd ever met, and she didn't believe any of the nonsense about how he was violent.

'He had completely charmed her.'

# Sources

1. Office for National Statistics, *Intimate personal violence and partner abuse* (2016). Available at www.ons.gov.uk/peoplepopulationandcommunity/crimeandjustice/compendium/focusonviolentcrimeandsexualoffences/yearendingmarch2015/chapter4intimatepersonalviolenceandpartnerabuse, accessed 10 February 2017.
2. Office for National Statistics, *Compendium Homicide* (2016) (average taken from last 10 years). Available at https://www.ons.gov.uk/peoplepopulationandcommunity/crimeandjustice/compendium/focusonviolentcrimeandsexualoffences/yearendingmarch2015/chapter2homicide, accessed 10 February 2017.
3. Fedders, C. and Elliott, L., *Shattered Dreams* (Harper & Row, 1987), p. 239.
4. Ibid. p. 48.
5. Polman, D., 'Judge closes the book on profits for wife abuser', *Chicago Tribune* (1988).
6. Walby, S., *The Cost of Domestic Violence* (Women and Equality Unit, 2004), p. 56. Available at http://www.devon.gov.uk/cost_of_dv_report_sept04.pdf, accessed 14 March 2017.
7. Lees, S., 'Marital Rape and Marital Murder', in J. Hanmer and N. Itzin (eds), *Home Truths about Domestic Violence: Feminist Influences on Policy and Practice: A Reader* (Routledge, 2000).
8. SafeLives, *Getting it right first time* (2015), p. 4. Available at www.safelives.org.uk/sites/default/files/resources/Getting%20it%20right%20first%20time%20executive%20summary.pdf, accessed 10 February 2017.
9. Her Majesty's Inspectorate of Constabulary (HMIC), *Crime-recording: Making the victim count* (2014), p.19. Available at www.justiceinspectorates.gov.uk/hmic/wp-content/uploads/crime-recording-making-the-victim-count.pdf, accessed 10 February 2017.
10. Taft, A., 'Violence against women in pregnancy and after childbirth: Current knowledge and issues in healthcare responses', *Australian Domestic and Family Violence Clearinghouse Issues*, Paper 6 (2002).
11. McFarlane, J. et al., 'Abuse during pregnancy and femicide: Urgent implications for women's health', *Obstetrics & Gynaecology* 100(1) (2002): pp. 27–36.
12. Sharp-Jeffs, N., *Money Matters* (London: Refuge / The Co-operative Bank, 2015). Available at www.refuge.org.uk/files/Money-Matters.pdf, accessed 8 January 2017.
13. SafeLives, *Who are the victims of domestic abuse?* Available at http://safelives.org.uk/policy-evidence/about-domestic-abuse/who-are-victims-domestic-abuse, accessed 8 January 2017.

14. Radford et al., *Child abuse and neglect in the UK today; Research into the prevalence of child maltreatment in the United Kingdom* (NSPCC, 2011). Available at https://www.nspcc.org.uk/services-and-resources/research-and-resources/pre-2013/child-abuse-and-neglect-in-the-uk-today/, accessed 14 March 2017.

15. Kincaid, P., *The Omitted Reality: Husband-wife Violence in Ontario and Policy Implications for Education* (1982).

16. Manning, V., *Estimates of the number of infants (under the age of one year) living with substance misusing parents* (NSPCC, 2011), p. 5. Available at https://www.nspcc.org.uk/globalassets/documents/research-reports/estimates-number-infants-living-with-substance-misusing-parents-report.pdf, accessed 12 February 2017.

17. Radford, L. et al., *Meeting the Needs of Children Living with Domestic Violence in London* (London: Refuge/NSPCC, 2011), pp. 100–05.

18. Aitken, R., *A Review of Children's Service Development (1995–1998) at Refuge* (Refuge/King's Fund, 1998) p. 17.

19. Women's Aid, *Child First Statistics*. Available at www.womensaid.org.uk/child-first-research, accessed 10 February 2017.

20. Women's Aid, *Nineteen Child Homicides* (Bristol: Women's Aid, 2016). Available at https://1q7dqy2unor827bqjls0c4rn-wpengine.netdna-ssl.com/wp-content/uploads/2016/01/Child-First-Nineteen-Child-Homicides-Report.pdf, accessed 10 February 2017.

21. Doward, J., 'Violent abusers to be prevented from cross-examining ex-partners in court', *The Guardian* (12 February 2017). Available at https://www.theguardian.com/law/2017/feb/12/domestic-violence-victims-get-help-in-prisons-bill, accessed 14 March 2017.

22. Humphreys, C. and Thiara, R., *Routes to Safety: Protection Issues Facing Abused Women and Children and the Role of Outreach Services* (Bristol: Policy Press, 2002).

23. Lees, S., 'Marital Rape and Marital Murder', in J. Hanmer and N. Itzin (eds), *Home Truths about Domestic Violence: Feminist Influences on Policy and Practice: A Reader* (Routledge, 2000).

24. Richards, L., *Findings from the Multi-agency Domestic Violence Murder Reviews in London* (Metropolitan Police, 2003). Available at http://www.dashriskchecklist.co.uk/wp-content/uploads/2016/09/Findings-from-the-Domestic-Homicide-Reviews.pdf, accessed 10 February 2017.

25. World Health Organization, *Violence against Women: Health Impact*. Available at www.who.int/reproductivehealth/publications/violence/VAW_health_impact.jpeg?ua=1, accessed 8 January 2017.

26. Walby, S., *The Cost of Domestic Violence* (Women and Equality Unit, 2004), p. 5. Available at www.devon.gov.uk/cost_of_dv_report_sept04.pdf, accessed 8 January 2017.

27. Johnson, J. M. and Ferraro, K. J., 'The Victimised Self: The Case of Battered Women', in J. A. Kotarba and A. Fortuna (eds), *The Existential Self in Society* (The University of Chicago Press, 1984), p. 120.

28. Ewing, C. P., *Battered Women Who Kill: Psychological Self-defense as Legal Justification* (Lexington Books, 1987), pp. 65–6.

29. Dutton, M. A., *Empowering and Healing the Battered Woman* (Springer Publishing Company, 1992).

30. Moss, K. and Singh, P., *70% of women rough sleepers have experienced domestic violence, research finds* (University of Wolverhampton, 2013). Available at https://www.wlv.ac.uk/about-us/news-and-events/latest-news/2013/january-2013/70-of-women-rough-sleepers-have-suffered-domestic-violence-research-finds.php, accessed 8 January 2017.

31. Kelly, L. and Dubois, L., *Combating Violence against Women: Minimum Standards for Support Services* (Directorate General of Human Rights and Legal Affairs, Council of Europe, 2008).

32. Women's Aid, *Why We Need to Save Our Services: Women's Aid Data Report on Specialist Domestic Violence Services in England* (Bristol: Women's Aid, 2014), p. 6.

33. Equality and Human Rights Commission, *Protecting Human Rights: Key Challenges for the UK's Third Universal Periodic Review* (September 2016), p.16.

34. Walker, L. E., *The Battered Woman* (Harper & Row, 1980).

35. Lifton, R. J., *Boundaries: Psychological Man in Revolution* (Vintage Books, 1969).

36. Her Majesty's Inspectorate of Constabulary (HMIC), *Everyone's Business: Improving the Police Response to Domestic Abuse* (2014), p. 5. Available at www.justiceinspectorates.gov.uk/hmic/wp-content/uploads/2014/04/improving-the-police-response-to-domestic-abuse.pdf, accessed 10 February 2017.

37. Ibid. p. 6.

38. Sanghani, R., 'Police officers admit calling alleged domestic abuse victim a "f****** slag" on voicemail', *The Telegraph* (2015). Available at www.telegraph.co.uk/women/womens-life/11957145/Domestic-violence-British-police-voicemail-called-victim-a-slag.html, accessed 10 February 2017.

39. Her Majesty's Inspectorate of Constabulary (HMIC), *PEEL: Police Legitimacy 2016, A National Overview* (2017), p. 33. Available at www.justiceinspectorates.gov.uk/hmic/wp-content/uploads/peel-police-legitimacy-2016.pdf, accessed 10 February 2017.

40. Walby, S. and Allen, J., *Domestic Violence, Sexual Assault and Stalking: Findings from the British Crime Survey* (London: Home Office Research, Development and Statistics Directorate, 2004).

41. Crown Prosecution Service, *Violence Against Women and Girls Crime Report 2015–16*, p. 5. Available at www.cps.gov.uk/news/latest_news/vawg_report_2016, accessed 10 February 2017.

42. Ibid.

43. Hall, A. (producer and director), *Behind Closed Doors* (BBC documentary, 2016). Available at www.youtube.com/watch?v=VvAoyh8UlEw, accessed 10 February 2017.

44. Tickle, L., 'Why is domestic abuse still not taken seriously in UK courts?', *The Guardian* (2016). Available at www.theguardian.com/society/2016/mar/08/

domestic-abuse-court-female-victims-bbc-documentary, accessed 10 February 2017.

45. Pizzey, E., *Prone to Violence* (1982), p. 72. Available at https://norskgoy.files. wordpress.com/2012/03/erinpizzey_pronetoviolence.pdf, accessed 10 February 2017.

46. Hester, M., *Who Does What to Whom? Gender and Domestic Violence Perpetrators* (University of Bristol, 2009). Available at http://www.nr-foundation.org.uk/ downloads/Who-Does-What-to-Whom.pdf p/9, accessed 14 March 2017.

47. Crown Prosecution Service, *Violence against Women and Girls Crime Report 2014–2015*, p. 15. Available at www.cps.gov.uk/publications/docs/cps_vawg_ report_2015_amended_september_2015_v2.pdf, accessed 8 January 2017.

48. Hester, M., *Who Does What to Whom? Gender and Domestic Violence Perpetrators* (University of Bristol, 2009). Available at www.nr-foundation. org.uk/downloads/Who-Does-What-to-Whom.pdf, accessed 8 January 2017.

49. Ansara, D. L. and Hindin, M. J., 'Psychosocial consequences of intimate partner violence for women and men in Canada', *Journal of Interpersonal Violence* 26(8) (2011): pp. 1628–45.

50. Radford, L. et al., *Meeting the Needs of Children Living with Domestic Violence in London* (London: Refuge/NSPCC, 2011), p. 104.

51. Sinclair, D., *Understanding Wife Assault: A Training Manual for Counsellors and Advocates* (Ontario Government Bookstore, 1985).

52. Ibid.

53. Equality and Human Rights Commission, *Protecting Human Rights: Key Challenges for the UK's Third Periodic Review* (2016), p. 19.

54. Women24, *Infographic: Marital rape is still legal in these 38 countries* (2016). Available at www.w24.co.za/Wellness/Mind/infographic-marital-rape-is-still-legal-in-these-38-countries-20151127, accessed 10 February 2017.

55. Marriage Foundation statistics, quoted in 'Marriage problems: More than a third of people are single or have never married', *The Guardian* (2015). Available at www.theguardian.com/lifeandstyle/2015/jul/08/record-number-england-wales-never-wed-marriage, accessed 8 January 2017.

56. Jenkin, M., 'Men still feel too embarrassed to ask for paternity leave', *The Guardian* (2015). Available at www.theguardian.com/sustainable-business/2015/oct/02/ paternity-leave-men-fathers-embarrassed-to-ask-for-parental-leave, accessed 8 January 2017.

57. Osborne, H., 'Tiny proportion of men are opting for shared parental leave', *The Guardian* (2016). Available at www.theguardian.com/money/2016/apr/05/ shared-parental-leave-slow-take-up-fathers-paternity, accessed 8 January 2017.

58. Equal Pay Portal, *Statistics* (2016). Available at www.equalpayportal.co.uk/ statistics, accessed 8 January 2017.

59. Ibid.

60. Toynbee, P., 'Never forget: half of absent fathers pay nothing towards raising their children', *The Guardian* (2015). Available at https://www.theguardian.com/commentisfree/2015/oct/15/half-absent-fathers-pay-nothing-alison-sharland-varsha-gohil, accessed 27 March 2017.

61. Department of Work and Pensions, *Child Support Agency Quarterly Summary of Statistics for Great Britain* (2016), p. 6.

62. Richardson, S., *Pamela* (Russell & Allen, 1811), pp. 409–11.

63. Mumsnet, *Chores: The Truth about Who Does What in the Modern Family* (2014). Available at www.mumsnet.com/surveys/chores-the-truth-about-who-does-what, accessed 10 February 2017.

64. Friar Cherubino, *The Rules of Marriage*, cited in M. L. McCue, *Domestic Violence: A Reference Handbook*, second edition (ABC-CLIO, 2008), p. 118.

65. Mill, J. S., *On Liberty with The Subjection of Women and Chapters on Socialism*, edited by Stefan Collini (Cambridge University Press, 1989), pp. 151–2.

66. Cobbe, F. P., 'Wife Torture in England', in S. Hamilton (ed.), *Criminals, Women, Idiots and Minors: Victorian Writing By Women On Women* (Broadview Press, 2004), p. 111.

67. Gratian, *Tractatus de Penetentia: A new Latin edition with English translation* (Catholic University of America Press, 2016).

68. Fedders, C. and Elliott, L., *Shattered Dreams* (Harper & Row, 1987), p. 5.

69. Byron, G. G., *Don Juan* (Galignani, 1831), p. 83.

70. Childs, S. and Campbell, R., 'This ludicrous obsession, parents in Parliament: The motherhood trap', *The Huffington Post* (2014). Available at www.huffingtonpost.co.uk/dr-rosie-campbell/women-in-politics_b_4608418.html, accessed 8 January 2017.

71. Campbell, R., quoted in H. Lewis, 'The motherhood trap', *New Statesman* (2015). Available at www.newstatesman.com/politics/2015/07/motherhood-trap, accessed 8 January 2017.

72. Bowcott, O., 'Proportion of female judges in UK among lowest in Europe', *The Guardian* (2016). Available at www.theguardian.com/law/2016/oct/06/proportion-of-women-judges-in-uk-among-lowest-in-europe, accessed 8 January 2017.

73. Coughlan, S., 'Why do women get more university places?' *BBC News* (2016). Available at www.bbc.co.uk/news/education-36266753, accessed 8 January 2017.

74. Hattenstone, S., 'Caroline Criado-Perez: Twitter has enabled people to behave in a way they wouldn't face to face', *The Guardian* (2013).

75. Bates, L., *Everyday Sexism*. Available at www.everydaysexism.com, accessed 10 February 2017.

76. McCabe, J. et al., 'Gender in twentieth-century children's books', *Gender and Society* 25(2) (2011), pp. 197–226. Summary available at www.theguardian.com/books/2011/may/06/gender-imbalance-children-s-literature, accessed 8 January 2017.

77.  Bridges, A. J. et al., 'Aggression and sexual behavior in best-selling pornography videos: A content analysis update', *Violence against Women* 16(10) (2010). Available at http://journals.sagepub.com/doi/abs/10.1177/1077801210382866, accessed 8 January 2017.

78.  Marshall, T., 'Nearly one third of rape victims are girls under 16', *London Evening Standard* (2016). Available at www.standard.co.uk/news/uk/nearly-one-third-of-rape-victims-are-girls-under-16-a3178641.html, accessed 10 February 2017.

79.  Rape Crisis England and Wales, *Statistics* (2017). Available at http://rapecrisis.org.uk/statistics.php, accessed 8 January 2017.

80.  Leo, B., 'Police scrap controversial rape prevention posters after criticism', *The Argus* (11 April 2015). Available at www.theargus.co.uk/news/12883974.Police_scrap_controversial_rape_prevention_posters_after_criticism, accessed 10 February 2017.

81.  Taaffe, H., *Sounds Familiar?* (The Fawcett Society, 2017). Available at www.fawcettsociety.org.uk/wp-content/uploads/2017/01/Sounds-Familiar-January-2017.pdf, accessed 10 February 2017.

82.  Office for National Statistics, *Compendium: Homicide* (2016). Available at www.ons.gov.uk/peoplepopulationandcommunity/crimeandjustice/compendium/focusonviolentcrimeandsexualoffences/yearendingmarch2015/chapter2homicide, accessed 8 January 2017.

83.  Yearnshire, S., 'Analysis of cohort', in S. Bewley, J. Friend, and G. Mezey, (eds), *Violence Against Women* (London: RCOG Press, 1997).

84.  Her Majesty's Inspectorate of Constabulary (HMIC), *PEEL: Police effectiveness 2016: A National Overview* (2017), Available at p.18 https://www.justiceinspectorates.gov.uk/hmic/wp-content/uploads/peel-police-effectiveness-2016.pdf, accessed 14 March 2017.

85.  Her Majesty's Inspectorate of Constabulary (HMIC), *Everyone's Business: Improving the Police Response to Domestic Abuse* (2014), p. 15. Available at www.justiceinspectorates.gov.uk/hmic/wp-content/uploads/2014/04/improving-the-police-response-to-domestic-abuse.pdf, accessed 10 February 2017.

86.  Pearmaine, E., *Police And Victims Urged To Use New Coercive Control Laws* (Simpson Millar LLP Solicitors, 2016). Available at www.simpsonmillar.co.uk/news/police-and-victims-urged-to-use-new-coercive-control-laws-3818, accessed 10 February 2017.

87.  Kelly, L. and Westmarland, N., *Domestic Violence Perpetrator Programmes: Steps Towards Change. Project Mirabal Final Report* (London Metropolitan University and Durham University, 2015), p. 18. Available at www.dur.ac.uk/resources/criva/ProjectMirabalfinalreport.pdf, accessed 8 January 2017.

88.  Ibid. p. 15.

89.  Ibid. p. 30.

90.  Ibid. p. 25.

91.  Home Office, *Guidance: Domestic Violence and Abuse* (2013). Available at www.gov.uk/guidance/domestic-violence-and-abuse, accessed 10 February 2017.

92. Home Office, *Domestic Homicide Reviews* (2016). Available at www.gov.uk/ government/uploads/system/uploads/attachment_data/file/575232/HO-Domestic-Homicide-Review-Analysis-161206.pdf, accessed 8 January 2017.
93. Walby, S., *The Cost of Domestic Violence: Up-date 2009* (Lancaster University, 2009).   Available   at   http://www.caadv.org.uk/new_cost_of_dv_2009.php, accessed 14 March 2017.

# Further Reading

Asher, R., *Shattered: Modern Motherhood and the Illusion of Equality* (Vintage, 2012).

Browne, A., *When Battered Women Kill* (New York Free Press, 1987).

Caplan, P., *The Myth of Women's Masochism* (E. P. Dutton, 1985).

Dutton, M. A., *Empowering and Healing the Battered Woman* (Springer Publishing Company, 1992).

Dworkin, A., *Our Blood* (The Women's Press, 1976).

Dworkin, A., *Pornography* (The Women's Press, 1982).

Edwards, S., *Policing 'Domestic Violence'* (Sage, 1989).

Halpern, H. M., *How to Break Your Addiction to a Person* (Bantam, 1982).

Hoffman, S., *Men Who Are Good For You and Men Who Are Bad* (Ten Speed Press, 1987).

Horley, S., *Love and Pain: A Survival Handbook for Women* (Bedford Square Press, 1988).

Lerner, H. G., *The Dance of Anger* (Harper & Row, 1985).

Martin, D., *Battered Wives* (Pocket Books, 1983).

NiCarthy, G., *Getting Free: A Handbook for Women in Abusive Relationships* (The Seal Press, 1982).

Russell, D. E. H., *Rape in Marriage* (Macmillan, 1982).

Russianoff, P., *Why Do I Think I Am Nothing Without a Man?* (Bantam, 1984).

Sanford, L. Tschirhart and Donovan, M. E., *Women and Self-Esteem* (Penguin, 1984).

Showalter, E., *The Female Malady: Women, Madness and English Culture, 1830–1980* (Virago, 1987).

Walker, L. E., *Terrifying Love* (Harper & Row, 1989).

Walker, L. E., *The Battered Woman* (Harper & Row, 1989).

Yllo, Kersti and Bogard, M., *Feminist Perspectives on Wife Abuse* (Sage, 1988).

# Useful Organisations

## Refuge

Refuge opened the world's first refuge in West London in 1971. Since then it has grown to become the country's largest provider of specialist domestic violence services. On any given day, Refuge is supporting almost 5,000 women and children who may have experienced domestic violence, rape and sexual assault, so-called 'honour'-based violence, female genital mutilation (FGM), forced marriage or modern slavery. Its services save and transform lives.

Refuge's services include:

- A national network of safe accommodation.
- Outreach projects, where staff work with women in the community.
- Independent domestic violence advocates, who provide expert guidance for women going through civil and criminal courts.
- Violence against women and girls (VAWG) services, which provide 'one-stop shops' where women who have experienced any form of gender-based violence can access a range of support.
- Culturally specific services, for women from Asian, Afro-Caribbean, Eastern European and Vietnamese backgrounds.
- Child support workers.
- The freephone 24-hour National Domestic Violence Helpline, run in partnership between Women's Aid and Refuge: 0808 2000 247.

# Other useful numbers

- **24/7 National Domestic Abuse and Forced Marriage Helpline Scotland, run by Scottish Women's Aid:** 0800 027 1234
- **24/7 Live Fear Free Helpline, run by Welsh Women's Aid:** 0808 80 10 800
- **Women's Aid Federation Northern Ireland, 24-hour Domestic & Sexual Violence Helpline:** 0808 802 1414
- **Women's Aid Ireland 24/7 National Freephone Helpline:** 1800 341 900
- **Samaritans:** 116 123
- **Rape Crisis:** 0808 802 9999
- **Shelter Housing Advice Helpline:** 0808 800 4444
- **Victim Support Free Helpline:** 0808 1689 111
- **Crimestoppers:** 0800 555 111

# Practical Guidance for Women

If you have recognised yourself or your partner in this book and you think you may be experiencing domestic abuse, you might be feeling confused, frightened or even ashamed. This is understandable, but the first thing to remember is: **you are not alone.** Refuge supports thousands of women like you every single day. Recognising you are being abused and deciding to get help is a brave and positive step; there are solutions to the problem, and Refuge is here to support you. Deciding what to do can take time. You may wish to involve the police, talk to Refuge, or end your relationship. Whatever you decide, your safety is always most important. And remember that **the abuse you have experienced is not your fault.**

Reaching out to Refuge:

- **Speak to an expert about your options** – you can speak to an adviser from the Freephone 24-hour National Domestic Violence Helpline, run in partnership by Refuge and Women's Aid, in confidence. The number to call is 0808 2000 247. They will be able to provide a listening ear for you to talk about your experiences as well as provide support to work through your options in the short and long term. The Helpline also acts as a 'gateway' to specialist domestic violence services throughout the country. The police and other agencies can also refer you to services.
- If you do not feel ready to phone the Helpline, you can visit **the Refuge website, www.refuge.org.uk** for support and information.

If you are still living with your abuser, think about how to protect yourself and your children:

- Be ready to call 999 if you or your children are in immediate danger.
- Make notes of abusive incidents, including times, dates, names and details of injuries – these can be important if you need to access legal and welfare rights.
- Keep some money and a set of keys in a safe place. For more information on preparing yourself financially to leave your partner, visit Refuge's My Money, My Life webpage.
- Find out about your legal and housing rights – talk to a solicitor if you can.
- Keep copies of important papers (passports, birth certificates, court orders, marriage certificate) in a safe place.
- Carry a list of emergency numbers: police, relatives, friends, the National Domestic Violence Helpline.
- Explore what civil or criminal options might be available to you, including restraining orders and injunctions such as non-molestation and occupation orders (which can ban a perpetrator from your home).
- Tell someone you trust about the abuse.
- Make calls from a phone box or a friend's house.
- Report any injuries to your GP so there is a record of the abuse.
- Talk to family and friends about staying with them in an emergency.
- Think about escape routes.

As hard as it might be when your partner is controlling and abusing you, try to find time to look after yourself if you can. Do something you enjoy. Taking time to read a book, walk in the park or listen to some music can help you feel more able to deal with what is happening. **Above all, remember that the abuse is not your fault.**

If you have left your partner, but are still in danger:

- Be ready to call 999 if you or your children are in immediate danger.
- Change the locks, and put locks on windows.
- Ask the police for advice about making your home more secure.
- Think about escape routes.
- Tell school who can pick up your children and who cannot.
- Report injuries to your GP so there is a record of the abuse.
- See a solicitor. They can make you aware of your rights and help you get a court order to protect you from your partner.

**If you would like to find out more about Refuge's work, or donate to the charity, visit www.refuge.org.uk or contact fundraising@ refuge.org.uk.**

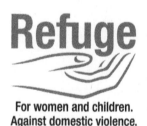

**For women and children.
Against domestic violence.**